The Health Planning Predicament

General Editor
CHARLES LESLIE

Editorial Board
FRED DUNN, M.D., University of California, San Francisco
RENÉE FOX, University of Pennsylvania
ELIOT FREIDSON, New York University
YASUO OTSUKA, M.D., Yokohama City University Medical School
CARL E. TAYLOR, M.D., The Johns Hopkins University
K. N. UDUPA, M.S., F.R.C.S., Banaras Hindu University
PAUL U. UNSCHULD, University of Munich
FRANCIS ZIMMERMANN, French Indological Institute

The Health Planning Predicament

Predicament

France, Québec, England, and the United States

VICTOR G. RODWIN

UNIVERSITY OF CALIFORNIA PRESS
Berkeley   Los Angeles   London

University of California Press
Berkeley and Los Angeles, California

University of California Press, Ltd.
London, England

Copyright © 1984 by
The Regents of the University of California

Library of Congress Cataloging in Publication Data

Rodwin, Victor G.
The health planning predicament.

(Comparative studies of health systems and medical care)
Includes bibliographical references and index.
1. Health planning—Case studies. I. Title.
II. Series. [DNLM: 1. Health planning.
WA 540.1 R697h]
RA393.R58 1983   362.1'0425   82-45910
ISBN 0-520-04445-2

Printed in the United States of America

1 2 3 4 5 6 7 8 9

For Lloyd and Nadine

CONTENTS

FOREWORD

From time to time a book appears that represents a fresh synthesis of a wide range of issues in a field. When this occurs, it may significantly reshape our ways of thinking. This is likely to be the case for Victor G. Rodwin's comparative analysis of health planning in France, the Canadian province of Québec, England, and the United States.

In examining the origins and recent evolution of health planning efforts, Victor Rodwin has probed deeply into the intricacies of the health care system in four different cultures. He has done this with great skill and sensitivity. There are several reasons why it has proved possible for him to do so. His professional training in economics, planning, and public health at the University of California, Berkeley, have grounded him in the theory, the methods, and the pragmatic concerns of these fields. In addition, he has traveled extensively and has taught courses on comparative health policy both at Berkeley and at the University of Paris-Dauphine. Before joining the faculty at the University of California, San Francisco, and developing a close association with the Institute for Health Policy Studies and the Aging Health Policy Center, Dr. Rodwin served as advisor to the Director of the French National Health Insurance Fund (CNAMTS). The insights he has garnered from his training and experience are evident in the scope and quality of this work.

Dr. Rodwin's focus is on France, Québec, and England. These countries have health systems with significant institutional differences and increasing degrees of state control over the organization and financing of health care—models toward which the United States is moving. France provides an example of a European national health insurance (NHI) system that covers both public and private hospitals as well as private practice on a fee-for-service basis. Québec provides another example of a NHI system; but unlike France and the other Canadian provinces, Québec represents a health system in which expanded state intervention has produced the most far-reaching institutional innovations undertaken to date in North America. England is the exemplar of a national health service (NHS): hospitals are controlled by the state and physicians are reimbursed on the basis of salaries and capitation fees.

Like other Western industrialized nations, in spite of the differences in organization and financing of their health care systems, France, Québec, and England share a set of common problems. First is the question of deciding what proportion of gross national product (GNP) should be devoted to health and welfare. Whether financing of health care expenditures is open-ended, as under NHI, or limited by budgetary allocations as under an NHS, there is always a problem of devising political and institutional mechanisms to decide on the government's financial contribution to the health sector. Second is the problem of agreeing on appropriate criteria to allocate health and social service expenditures. In France, Québec, and England, health planners agree that poor coordination between hospitals and community based services has resulted in excessive reliance on hospital care for services that could best be provided in other institutions or in the community—for example, long-term care for the elderly. Third is the problem of how to implement established policies: through regulation, promotion of competition, budgeting, or reimbursement of hospitals and physicians.

Any attempt to sum up the main ideas of such a wide-ranging study risks being misleading. But there are two points, in particular, which we are inclined to emphasize—probably because we strongly agree with them. The first point is technical; the second is sociopolitical.

The technical point involves the need for government to link and control the planning and financing of health care services. Dr. Rodwin carefully documents the ways in which these functions remain separate not only in the United States but in France, Québec, and England, as well. He suggests that the failure to link planning criteria to health care financing is the "Achilles' heel of contemporary health planning practice." What are the implications of this analysis for health policy in the United States? Clearly, there will have to be changes in our predominant mechanisms of provider reimbursement.

The Reagan Administration is currently dismantling the formal health planning program mandated by P.L. 93-641 while encouraging significant change in Medicare and Medicaid reimbursement policies and attempting to stimulate competition in the health sector. At the same time, new coalitions of business interests are promoting efforts at cost control. But such efforts are now being pursued at the expense of the very poor and disadvantaged. There are no longer participatory planning mechanisms in the health sector to protect the public interest. Whether health planning strategies rely on regulation, competition or, what Rodwin calls "regulated competition," there is no way to escape the critical policy issue raised by the idea of linking health planning and health care financing: how to design a reimbursement system that would encourage hospitals and physicians to pursue society's interest as well as their own?

The sociopolitical point involves the obstacles in the way of creating effective linkages between representative health planning bodies and the institutions that control health care financing: payers, rate setters, and budgetary authorities. The fact is that there are powerful groups in all countries who are in a strategic position to manipulate the system to serve their interests and who see no advantages in having democratic, often participatory planning bodies, alter the existing allocation of health resources. The sociopolitical obstacles to implementation of health planning goals involve not only opposition of vested interests such as organized medicine but also deep differences in political philosophy. As Dr. Rodwin notes in his chapter on the role of the state in health care (chap. 2), even liberals who unlike conservatives and radicals think the state can cope with the problems of the health sector, concede that the difficulties are formidable.

Whether or not one agrees with these and other conclusions of Victor Rodwin, this book is bound to provoke spirited and fruitful discussion and it is likely to broaden the debate about the state of health planning today.

Philip R. Lee, M.D.
Professor of Social Medicine
Director, Institute for Health Policy Studies
University of California, San Francisco

Carroll L. Estes, Ph.D.
Professor of Sociology
Director, Aging Health Policy Center
University of California, San Francisco

PART I
INTRODUCTION

1

THE NATURE OF
HEALTH PLANNING

Since World War II, Western industrial nations have created institutions to plan for health care services. This has led to a demand for specialists to address issues of health planning. Health planners may be government administrators, corporate managers, policy analysts, civil servants, or health professionals. The one distinguishing characteristic they share is a concern with some basic health care issues: How should a health care system be organized and financed to meet the needs of the public? What is the appropriate role of hospitals? What are appropriate responsibilities for preventive medicine and for public health programs? How can health care needs be assessed to answer these questions? How should providers of health care (hospitals and physicians) be reimbursed?

Until the mid-1960s, health planners focused on the problems of managing growth. Their goals were clear—to eliminate financial barriers to medical care, to reduce the gap between new biomedical knowledge and its practical applications and availability and, above all, to build and modernize hospitals. There was widespread agreement about these goals and they were largely accomplished. Physicians, hospitals, and consumers all benefited—more or less—from what has come to be known as the "medical-industrial complex."[1]

Over the past decade, the character of the problems, the context of planning, and the goals have changed. The new problems paradoxically are a result of previous success. The reduction of financial barriers to medical care, the greater availability of new medical technology, and the growth of hospitals dramatized the problems of inequitable access to services and resulted in rapid escalation of health care costs. Health planners have turned their attention to the task of managing retrenchment.

In addition to these problems, growth of the health professions and new claims on health resources by citizens and organized interest groups have turned the health sector into a major political arena. The number of physicians has grown and the degree of specialization has increased. This has fractured the unity that once prevailed in the medical profession and has reinforced hierarchy. At the same time, new actors such as paraprofessionals, labor unions, the biomedical research establishment, and consumer representatives participate in health planning efforts. As a result of these changes, the principal interest groups no longer agree on what goals to pursue.

The goals of health planning have broadened. There is a growing emphasis, today, on the design of new institutions for providing health care, the pursuit of health promotion campaigns, and the need for rationalization, that is, for securing a more efficient allocation of resources in the health sector. In the context of rising health care costs and growing conflict over issues of resource allocation, health planners face a predicament. No one quite knows what the future health sector should look like or how to gain control over the health care system.

TWO IMAGES OF HEALTH PLANNING

Health planners typically view rationalization as the goal of redistributing health resources away from hospital-centered care to public health programs and community based health and social services. In contrast, political economists and social historians view rationalization as a process of social transformation—of adapting anachronistic institutions to the exigencies of a changing economy. For example, Stephen Cohen and Charles Goldfinger characterize such "chronic adaptation" in the service sector as a kind of "permacrisis";[2] Larry Hirshhorn views it as a phase of "disaccumulationist capitalism";[3] and James Weinstein sees rationalization as a strategy by corporate interests to reform the institutional structure.[4]

Two traditions underlie these seemingly different views of rationalization: one is that of social reform; the other is that of systems maintenance. The tradition of social reform is utopian: it seeks to achieve equality and to redress social and economic injustices. The tradition of systems maintenance is conservative: it seeks to preserve the status quo and to overcome obstacles to economic stability. Most of the key issues in the literature on planning can be subsumed under one or another of these traditions. Both social reform and systems maintenance involve what Karl Mannheim called "societal guidance."[5] And both can converge, as they did in the United States during the progressive era and the New Deal.

Henrik Blum's image of health planning as "deliberate social change" is a prime example of the social reformist tradition.[6] Most health planners, he suggests, follow some variation of the sequential planning process steps outlined in figure 1. These activities, he adds, may take place at the different levels indicated in figure 2, which range from belief systems and national policy to specific legislative bills and service delivery units.

Other scholars in the field of health planning have a quite different image of their subject. They focus less on the kind of planning undertaken and more on who does the planning and whose interests it serves. They are concerned with how deliberate social change is controlled by corporate interests to reinforce the "regulatory reproduction of the status quo."[7] For example, Elliott Krause, in his analysis of

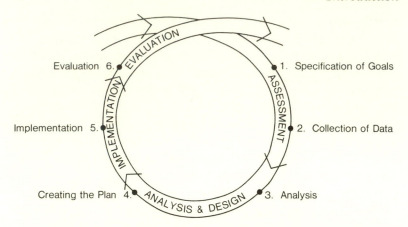

Fig. 1. Elements of the health planning process.

Source: Adapted from Henrik Blum, *Planning for Health*, 2d ed. (New York: Human Services Press, 1981), p. 54.

major federal health programs in the United States, argues that the planning process does not produce social reform, rather it reinforces the existing status quo within the health sector.[8] Robert Alford arrives at similar conclusions based on a study of health care reform in New York. He laments, "The very mechanisms which are intended to insure planning guarantee that no planning takes place. The very mechanisms of coordination become instruments of the status quo."[9]

DOCTRINAL CONTROVERSIES IN PLANNING

There is discord in professional circles on the meaning of planning. This has led Aaron Wildavsky to insist that "If Planning is Everything," (future control, cause, power, adaptation, process, intention, rationality, faith)—"Maybe It's Nothing!"[10] But is planning everything?

Planning is most often conceived of in contrast to free market behavior. In theory, the market allows for multiple

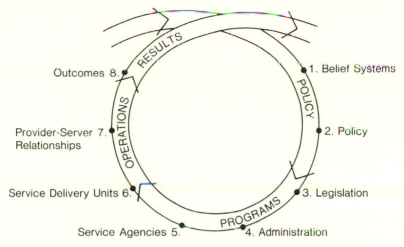

Fig. 2. Levels of Planning for Social Change

Source: Adapted from Henrik Blum, *Planning for Health*, 2d ed. (New York: Human Sciences Press, 1981), p. 52.

individual decisions. It requires only limited state intervention and it results in a system in which price information is readily available. Resources move in response to price signals and there is a complementary public sector in which collective "nonmarket goods" are produced. In contrast, when planning replaces the market, Stephen Cohen observes,

> Shaping the future of society passes from a process of causation to a process of decision. At present, the direction of development is "caused"; it is not decided. In a market system the shape of development is caused by complex interactions of countless decisions that are all taken without any concern as to the shape of the whole; the pattern of development is an unintended outcome. Pragmatic politics enters the causation process in disjointed piecemeal fashion to temper and to steer it a bit. But it does not substitute an alternative process of deliberate decision for the present process of unplanned causation.[11]

Despite this plausible distinction between planning and market, there is still controversy over just what planning entails. For some, planning means replacing the market with a Kafkaesque public bureaucracy charged with designing regulations. For others, this is a worst case caricature. They emphasize instead that planning aids the market by anticipating future problems and improving information for making decisions. For still others, planning involves stabilization policy; and others see it as a process of setting social priorities by creating systematic processes of social diagnosis, policy analysis, decision making, and evaluation.

Melvin Webber suggests that planning is essentially a way of thinking, a cognitive style, "that process of making rational decisions about future goals and future courses of action which relies upon explicit tracings of the repercussions and of the value implications associated with alternative courses of actions, and in turn requires explicit evaluation and choice among alternative matching goal-action sets."[12] John Forester associates this style with the relationships between analysis and design. Planners, he says, are involved not merely in problem solving and in applying social science to social problems but also are concerned with problem finding, that is to say, with mobilizing attention to practical questions that matter.[13]

Others stress the roles of planners in forecasting, innovating, scheduling, implementing, negotiating, and coalition building as well as in preparing plans. Aaron Wildavsky goes even further. He observes (what planners discerned much earlier) that "there does not have to be a plan to have planning. Any process of decision that affects behavior, whether market or administrative, may be thought of as a plan insofar as it provides incentives for generating one sort of future behavior rather than another."[14]

At the opposite extreme, in an analysis of "centrally planned change," James Q. Wilson views planning as a process of central control. He suggests that a system with decentralization of formal authority, participation, and pluralism puts a high value on consensus and therefore usually blocks efforts at central planning. He concludes ironically that "each temporary success at central planning will eventually elicit the opposition of the planning profession, for the political terms upon which planning is possible at all in America are typically terms that lead to plans that displease the defenders of planning."[15] Wilson adds that the terms are such in the United States that change must proceed on an incremental basis, "not simply because there are systematic biases against change but also . . . because most actors on the scene prefer it that way."[16]

Unfortunately, Wilson does not investigate the broader forces that produce not only incremental change but also big, structural change of the kind that has occurred in the industrial sector (steel and automobiles) as well as in the health sector. Where Wilson concludes his analysis of central planning is where one ought to begin raising questions about the nature of planning. For the crucial issues—at least as far as this study is concerned—are not whether central planning exists, or whether there should be more or less planning as opposed to the market. Rather, once one acknowledges the existence of planning—if not some idealized version, then at least in the form of systematic state intervention in the economy—it is important to distinguish different kinds of planning and to understand their essential characteristics.

By distinguishing between different kinds of health planning, it may be possible to learn why some kinds of planning do work and some do not and why some planners are displeased with the kind of planning that does work. To understand the field of planning, however, it seems more fruitful to examine what its practitioners do, not what theorists say they do. Indeed, that is the most important task of this study—to assess what health planners have actually done; what they are now doing in different national environments; and what this means for the United States and for health planning efforts, in general.

THE PLAN AND THEMES OF THIS STUDY

In the field of planning and policy studies, we are often ethnocentric in our perspectives. For this reason, the core of this book consists of case studies of health planning efforts abroad: in France, in the Canadian province of Québec, and in England.* Each case analyzes the sociopolitical and historical context within which planning operates. Each also evaluates the country's experience with respect to two overlapping criteria of plan implementation: (1) the extent to which particular kinds of health planning succeeded in terms of their stated goals, and (2) the extent to which health planners succeeded in altering the allocation of health resources in line with their plans.[17]

Windows can sometimes be mirrors. A look at health planning abroad can reflect insights about efforts to plan for health services at home. Thus, following the case studies, I evaluate the experience of health planning in the United States from the perspective of what can be learned from health planning efforts abroad (chap. 8). I also examine the current debate about whether to dismantle the formal health planning system and replace it by a system that encourages competition in the health sector.

As a preface to the case studies, I provide an overview of each health care system (chap. 4), including that of the United States (to make explicit the standard of comparison). I examine, first, the broad institutional setting; next, the financing and organization of medical care; finally, the reimbursement incentives that influence the behavior of medical care providers.

The French experience with health planning (chap. 5) provides a paradigmatic model of health sector rationaliza-

---

*Much of what is said about Québec and England applies as well to Canada and the United Kingdom. Nonetheless, I focus on Québec and England because there is significant variation between the health policies of Canadian provinces and between the constituent nations of the United Kingdom (England, Wales, Scotland, and Northern Ireland).

tion. Growth of health expenditures in France increased fiscal and parafiscal pressures (from income and payroll taxes) and raised the production costs of industry. Production costs get passed down to consumers either through real wage losses or price increases. Both are politically unacceptable. Price increases, in particular, place French firms at a competitive disadvantage in the European Economic Community; and this runs counter to the stated objectives of the national economic plan and to the interests of big business and the ministry of finance. Thus, the experience of France illustrates how the process of rationalizing the health sector involves a political battle to keep rising costs under control in an environment of increasing social demands on health insurance and fierce resistance by professional interests.

The experience with health planning in Québec (chap. 6), points up two phases of rationalization. During the so-called quiet revolution of the sixties, while the Liberal party was in power, health planning served as an instrument for broadening the scope of medical care to include proposals for comprehensive reform of the welfare and social service sectors. Subsequently, the process of legislating major health care reforms led to confrontation between physicians, community representatives, and the provincial government. The broad goals of institutional renovation were soon compromised by political and economic constraints.

The English experience with health planning (chap. 7), illustrates two other variations of rationalization. First, health planners attempted to eliminate the inherited tripartite structure of the national health service which separated the administration of public health services from that of hospital and primary-care services. This effort resulted in a new formal planning system for the NHS and a reorganized administrative structure that aimed to streamline management and increase central control. Next, health planners in England took advantage of the special opportunities offered by a national health service to make implicit trade-offs in the resource allocation process explicit and thereby pave the way for explicit health care rationing. England, a laggard in hospital construction and modernization, became a forerunner in the process of health sector rationalization.

There is a common theme in these case studies as well as in the chapter on health planning in the United States (chap. 8). It is that health planning efforts aimed at rationalization—in contrast to the earlier efforts aimed at managing growth—have encountered formidable obstacles. Critical elements of plans have not been implemented. One important reason is that health planning is not effectively linked to health care financing, particularly to reimbursement incentives and budgeting mechanisms that influence medical care providers. But there are other reasons why implementation is difficult to achieve. These include: (1) the limited applicability of modern management techniques to problems in the health sector; (2) resistance to change by professional interests; and (3) systemic constraints on state intervention in a capitalist economy. In the final chapter (chap. 9), I summarize the experience with health planning in all four countries, examine these barriers to implementation in more detail, and speculate about the impact of emerging trends on health planning.

There is unavoidably some implicit theorizing that comes with telling the story of health planning in each country. This is why I make the ideas and assumptions of this study more explicit in the two chapters that follow. To begin with, I explain why health planning efforts have emerged in Western industrial nations. This leads to a discussion of three contrasting perspectives on the role of the state in society and their implications for health planning (chap. 2). Next, I focus on the technical dimensions of the health planning predicament: setting standards for the proper allocation of health resources and securing implementation of plans. Based on some propositions about the nature of the medical care system in the United States, I suggest that to achieve control over the allocation of health resources it is necessary to link health planning activities to the institutions that finance health care (chap. 3).

PART II
BACKGROUND AND APPROACH

2

HEALTH PLANNING
AND THE STATE

One of the more remarkable changes over the last half-century in industrially advanced nations has been the trend toward more systematic state intervention in the form of national economic planning. In socialist nations such as the Soviet Union, the revolution produced rapid social transformation and the market mechanism was replaced by a system of national economic planning. In Western capitalist nations such as Canada, France, and Great Britain, despite the absence of revolution throughout the twentieth century, there have also been rapid social and economic changes resulting in the growth of the state and the emergence of national planning institutions. Ironically, in socialist nations greater reliance on the market has been justified in order to refine the practice of planning, whereas in capitalist nations, national economic planning has most often been justified as a way to correct market failures.

In Western capitalist nations, as the state's role in financing health care has expanded, policymakers have tried to promote the efficiency and equity of public expenditures. Budget deficits at all levels of government, the taxpayer revolt, and pressure from business to maintain a favorable environment for investments have forced governments to cut back public expenditures and rationalize public services to promote a more efficient allocation of resources. Just as economic planning in Europe was a response to common changes in the economies of industrially advanced nations, so too have health planning efforts been a response to structural change both within and outside the health sector and to common problems resulting from health sector growth.

There are three main perspectives in political economy, which help understand controversy about the proper role of the state in the health sector. Conservatives oppose state intervention, in general, and health planning, in particular, and support increased reliance either on professionalism or on entrepreneurial (free enterprise) medicine. Radicals oppose state intervention under existing institutional arrangements and support either socialized medicine or deprofessionalized medicine. Liberals justify an incremental ameliorative role for state intervention and support health planning efforts on grounds of rationality, equity, and accountability. This chapter interprets the emergence of health planning, summarizes these perspectives on the role of the state, and explores their implications for health planning.

HEALTH PLANNING AS A RESPONSE TO CHANGE

PATTERNS OF CHANGE OUTSIDE THE HEALTH SECTOR

Andrew Shonfield discerns five changes that converted capitalism from the cataclysmic failure of the thirties to a great "engine of prosperity" in the sixties:[1]

1. The increasing influence of public authorities in economic management made possible by the increase of state expenditures.
2. The new and widely shared assumption among policymakers that each year should bring an increase in per capita real income.

3. The increased regulation and control of competition to tame the "violence of the market."
4. The increased level of social welfare, particularly expenditures for health, education, and pensions.
5. Finally, the emergence of new attitudes concerning large-scale economic management both inside government and in the private sector; the concern for intellectual coherence, long range planning, or as Pierre Massé called it, "l'anti-hasard."[2]

In retrospect, after a decade of lower growth rates and fiscal crisis, as well as the energy crises of 1973 and 1979, Shonfield appears prematurely optimistic. But, whether one is inclined to praise capitalism or to denounce it, it requires ideological stamina to deny that modern capitalism is moving toward increased state control and planning.[3] In addition to the pressures pushing toward national planning, modern capitalism as well as Soviet socialism are being transformed by an accelerated growth of new technology and by a massive shift in occupational structure. Whereas the industrial revolution swept peasants off the land and into factories, the so-called postindustrial revolution is characterized by the growth of service as opposed to goods-producing industries.[4] Health, education, welfare, and administration, both public and private, have become the new sectors for employment growth.

GROWTH AND CHANGE WITHIN THE HEALTH SECTOR

Since World War II, the most striking characteristic of the health sector in industrially advanced nations has been its explosive growth. There has been an extraordinary burgeoning of health sector employment, of health care utilization, and of health care costs. The health sector has responded to powerful new forces: changes in the *demand* for health care and changes in the *supply* structure of health care.

On the demand side, a number of factors account for the increasing utilization of health services. First, rapid economic growth has increased per capita real income. For example, in the United States, between 1950 and 1973, per capita disposable income increased by 76 percent (in constant 1958 dollars).[5] More disposable income means more money to spend on health services; and, indeed, the money has been spent.

In addition to private affluence, the state has become involved in the financing of health care. As medical technology has brought new diagnostic and therapeutic procedures, they have been covered under health insurance programs and have contributed to increasing the use of medical services. As social problems have become increasingly "medicalized" (e.g., alcoholism treatment services and long-term care for the elderly), these have also been covered under health insurance.[6]

Another factor that accounts for the increasing use of health services is the demographic change in industrially advanced nations. Increased life expectancy at birth and declining birthrates have greatly increased the percentage of the population that is over sixty-five years old. Since the elderly suffer from illness and disability more often than younger people, they tend to visit physicians more frequently and have higher hospital admission rates. Still other factors that account for the increasing use of health services are the change in patterns of disease and the growth of medical technology. The major health problems in industrially advanced nations are no longer infectious diseases but chronic degenerative conditions, such as cardiovascular disease, cancer, and arthritis. This is partly owing to the increased percentage of elderly in the population but it also reflects broader changes in industrial society and the social effects of economic growth and technological progress. For example, automobile accidents have increased the number and severity of emergency room cases. Further, the availability of new diagnostic procedures and therapies has led physicians to increase the range and quantity of medical procedures prescribed.

Finally, demand for health services has increased because of changes in socioeconomic characteristics: for example, changes in occupational structure—more white-collar and professionally trained workers; in level of education—more public information on the potential benefits of health care; and in geographic location—more people living in cities. These factors are closely correlated among themselves and with high utilization of health services. They are a reminder of how much the activities in the health sector are dependent upon the socioeconomic system of which they are a part. After all, the health sector is financed, for the most part, out of collective funds—government, Social Security, and private insurance. It relies on the educational system for producing increasing numbers of diversified and highly skilled professionals, and it receives its patients according to the social system's changing and broader definitions of health.

On the supply side, there are also a number of factors that account for health sector growth. Growth of biomedical knowledge, innovations in medical technology, and increasing medical specialization have transformed traditional medical practice; and they continue to transform the structure of health services in nations throughout the world. The health sector has grown from a sort of "cottage industry" composed of entrepreneurial physicians providing most of their services in the patient's home to a major industrial complex centered in highly specialized hospitals and supporting significant affiliated activities such as the pharmaceutical industry, biomedical testing laboratories, and firms producing and marketing medical technology.

Since the beginning of this century, the hospital has been transformed from a largely philanthropic institution caring for (and sometimes experimenting on) the indigent sick to a center supplied with basic medical infrastructure performing the highest functions of the health system—teaching,

basic research, and diagnosis and therapy of complex illnesses. The growth of biomedical knowledge and medical
technology has brought a new corps of medical specialists,
technicians, and paraprofessionals into the health sector,
thus increasing the division of labor and hierarchy.

The organization of primary care has not been immune
to these changes. The country doctor isolated in solo practice with longstanding clients is gradually receding behind
new forms of collective and, often, salaried practice. Networks tying together practitioners with infrastructure or
support services, group practice, and health and social service centers have emerged as new organizational settings for
the delivery of ambulatory care. Other modes of health care
delivery are rapidly being developed, such as health maintenance organizations (HMOs), home health care programs, one-day hospital procedures, and such preventive
health programs as occupational health and safety, maternal and child health, and blood pressure screening.

PARADOXES OF HEALTH SECTOR GROWTH

One might expect that the growth of the health sector
would lead to improved health status and access to medical
care. Paradoxically, however, there have been negative side
effects and new problems accompanying this growth.

Despite the abundance of medical services in industrially
advanced nations, it is by no means evident that more medical care produces a healthier population.[7] Moreover, the
evidence in the United States suggests that despite the increased use of medical services by the poor since 1965, the
disparity in life expectancy between upper and lower classes
has increased over the past decade.[8] Despite therapeutic
innovations that have become a symbol of medical progress,
two unsuspected problems have emerged: the marginal
effectiveness of many technologically advanced therapies
and the increasing incidence of iatrogenic, that is, medically
induced, disease.

Another side effect of health sector growth is that disparities in the distribution of health resources are exacerbated by progress in medical technology for innovation is more readily adopted by the more urbanized areas and privileged groups. As a consequence, despite the increased use of medical services, the geographic distribution of specialty care has become more inequitable. In the United States, financial barriers to access still exist, not only for those without health insurance but also for health insurance subscribers who pay substantial deductibles and copayments. In the Soviet Union and England, although access to primary care has been generalized to the entire population, access to elective or specialty services may depend on party connections (USSR), ability to tolerate queues (England), or ability to pay private sector prices (both USSR and England).

In addition to exacerbating the problem of differential access to health services, health sector growth has resulted in rising health care costs. In the United States, for example, employee benefits for health and life insurance increased by 1,731 percent between 1951 and 1979, while the consumer price index increased by only 190 percent.[9] A recent study by the Organization for Economic Cooperation and Development (OECD) indicates that public expenditures on health, as a proportion of gross domestic product (GDP), increased by an average of almost 2 percent from 1962 to 1974 for all OECD countries (table 1). This rate of growth is significantly more than the increase of public expenditures on education and income maintenance.[10] In 1980 total health expenditures rose to as high as 9.6 percent of GDP in the United States to 8.1 percent in France, 7.4 percent in Canada, and 5.7 percent in the United Kingdom.[11]

THE ROLE OF THE STATE: CONTRASTING PERSPECTIVES

The state has gradually expanded its role in the health sector. Its responsibility has grown from enforcing minimal

Background and Approach

TABLE 1
CHANGES IN CURRENT EXPENDITURE ON HEALTH,
1962 TO 1974 OR NEAR DATES

	Changes in shares in "trend" GDP (percentage points)	
Country	Total expenditure on health	Public expenditure on health
Australia (FY 1962–1975)	1.7	2.5
Austria*	1.1	.8
Belgium (1965–1974)	.7	1.1
Canada (1962–1973)	1.6	2.6
Denmark	–	2.7
Finland (1962–1975)	1.9	3.0
France	2.2	2.2
Germany (1960–1974)	2.2	2.7
Ireland (1963–1975)	2.4	2.6
Italy	2.1	2.3
Japan (1960–1975)	1.1	1.6
Netherlands (1963–1972)	2.9	2.3
New Zealand (FY 1961–1974)	1.1	.9
Norway (1962–1973)	2.3	2.9
Sweden (1963–1974)	2.6	3.1
Switzerland (1960–1973)	1.2	1.5
United Kingdom (1962–1975)	1.3	1.4
United States (1960–1974)	2.4	1.8

Source: Adapted from table 11 in *Public Expenditure on Health* (Paris: OECD Studies in Resource Allocation, July, 1977).
*Percentage points for countries not followed by parentheses refer to period from 1962–1974.

sanitary conditions and running public health programs to financing medical care, regulating the growth of the health sector, reorganizing health care institutions, and, in some cases, assuming even more control over the health sector through nationalization (in England) or socialization (in the Soviet Union).

We know that the growing involvement of the state in matters of health provokes intense reactions. It is also generally accepted that the basic subject matter and modes of analysis in the study of social policy are informed by an "interpretation of beliefs" that, by its nature, is not susceptible to rigorous tests.[12] This phenomenon is not a frailty of social science; it is a fundamental condition that affects our views in all fields, including the physical sciences.[13]

What presuppositions or interpretations of beliefs affect our views on the proper role of the state in society? We will summarize three orienting perspectives crudely identified as conservative, radical, and liberal.[14] Although they are well known, they are seldom explicitly articulated. For those trained in moral philosophy and political theory, these perspectives will seem like a caricature. But even in this form they are helpful in coming to grips with the powerful ideological undercurrents in health planning.

THE CONSERVATIVE PERSPECTIVE

Conservative beliefs may be traced to British social and political thought ranging from the traditionalist views of Edmund Burke to certain strands of the economic and political liberalism of Adam Smith and John Stuart Mill.[15] Above all, conservatives believe in the importance of social order and authority. Because they respect the wisdom of the past as embodied in existing institutions, they believe that social change should proceed slowly especially when little is known about the consequences. Conservatives categorically reject utopian solutions to human problems.

A number of contemporary conservative beliefs are expressed today in the writings of Milton Friedman. His underlying values are libertarian since he emphasizes the social value of personal responsibility for achievement and maximum individual freedom. Such values emerge clearly, for example, in Friedman's vision of the ideal society: "unanimity among responsible individuals achieved on the basis of free and full discussion. . . . The ultimate end is itself the use of the proper means."[16]

In practice, of course, unanimity among individuals is rare. Thus, Friedman accepts a political system based on majority rule. Most decisions, in his view, should be made by individuals through "voluntary exchange" in the context of a free market. Friedman claims that consumers should be sovereign because they know better than anyone else, their own preferences. He warns about the need to limit strictly the coercive power of the state and he likens the ideal role of the state to that of an umpire and rule-maker. To Friedman, the state is somehow above society—neutral—and charged with mediating the multiple demands of competing interest groups. In his essay, "The Role of Government in a Free Society," Friedman emphasizes that

> the organization of economic activity through voluntary exchange presumes that we have provided, through government, for the maintenance of law and order to prevent coercion of one individual by another, the enforcement of contracts voluntarily entered into, the definition of the meaning of property rights, the interpretation and enforcement of such rights, and the provision of a monetary framework.[17]

Beyond these general functions for the government, Friedman supports state intervention only in the presence of natural monopolies and externalities. In the case of natural monopolies where it is technically efficient to have only one producer, he is prepared to choose between the evils of private monopoly, public monopoly, or public regulation. In the case of externalities, when the voluntary exchange of goods and services does not obey the "exclusion principle," that is when the actions of individuals have side effects on third parties for which it is impossible to recompensate them (e.g., pollution), Friedman is willing to consider the possibility of government intervention. But he does this reluctantly, because in his view "every act of government intervention limits the area of individual freedom directly and threatens the preservation of freedom indirectly."[18]

Radicals and liberals hold that equality promotes fraternal bonds and consequently assures greater social stability. Conservatives hold that people are, by nature, unequal and that state intervention to achieve equality threatens personal freedom and weakens those economic incentives needed to promote economic growth: *in dubito, cum statu quo.*

THE RADICAL PERSPECTIVE

Radical beliefs are rooted in the nineteenth-century Hegelian-Marxist tradition. With respect to freedom and personal responsibility for achievement, radicals turn their attention away from the individual and emphasize the social. Conservatives define freedom as the absence of restraint; radicals understand freedom as collective self-determination. Radicals argue that freedom and human development can be realized only if social inequalities are reduced. Whereas analysts who hold conservative beliefs emphasize *equality under the law* and those who hold liberal beliefs advocate *equality of opportunity*, analysts with radical beliefs tend to promote *equality of results*.

Like the conservative perspective, the radical one also has its ideal: a classless, cooperative society in which private property is abolished, exploitation is eliminated, and individual autonomy and potential is realized. This is communism. In practice, since the idea is far from being realized, contemporary radicals have concentrated on analyzing the problems of the modern capitalist state.[19] They reject what Paul Sweezy calls the "class-mediation" theory of the state,

the tendency on the part of modern liberal theorists to interpret the state as an institution established in the interests of society as a whole for the purpose of mediating and reconciling the antagonisms to which social existence inevitably gives rise. . . . The class-mediation theory assumes, usually implicitly, that the underlying class structure, or what comes to the same thing, the system of property relations, is an immutable datum.[20]

Radicals emphasize and view the system from a historical perspective. They see property relations as the outcome of class struggle. Thus, they are more sympathetic to "class domination" theories of the state. Instrumentalist theorists of the state such as Miliband elaborate on the proposition by Marx and Engels that "the modern state is but a committee for managing the common affairs of the whole bourgeoisie."[21] Structuralist theorists of the state such as Poulantzas reject the interpretation of the capitalist state as an instrument of the ruling class and emphasize the "objective" functions of state intervention within a capitalist economy. More recent scholars sharing radical perspectives attempt to transcend these categories.

Habermas, for example, criticizes the modern capitalist state as heading toward a crisis of legitimacy.[22] In analyzing the need for the "accumulation-supporting state" to legitimate itself before the electorate, Habermas distinguishes several kinds of rationality. He explains how increasing societal demands on the state combined with limited intellectual, ideological, and organizational resources lead to "rationality deficits."

In contrast, O'Connor proposes a three sector model of the capitalist economy: the monopoly sector, the competitive sector, and the state sector. He explores the contradiction between the requirements of the state for expanded revenues and the maintenance of capital accumulation. Also, he shows how accumulation and legitimation lead to demands for greater state expenditure; hence, the "fiscal crisis of the state."[23]

Probably the most innovative radical perspective on the theory of the state is Claus Offe's recent work on the "internal structure" of the state and its role in policy formation. He argues that the capitalist state has four principal attributes: (1) It is *excluded* from ordering and controlling production because enterprises are free. (2) It must deflect threats to accumulating units and *maintain* the conditions for capital accumulation. (3) In order to raise revenues and meet its obligations the state *depends* on the accumulating units for its own stability. (4) Faced with the unstable functions of *exclusion, maintenance,* and *dependency,* it seeks to "convey the image of an organization of power that pursues common and general interests of society as a whole, allows equal access to power and is responsive to justified *demands*"—legitimation.[24]

Offe goes on to consider the character of state production. He distinguishes *allocative* from *productive* policies. Offe first formulates "decision rules" for the process of policy formation; then he indicates how the mechanisms necessary to maintain the structural attributes of the capitalist state change as capitalism evolves: as the capitalist state increasingly pursues "productive policies" (state production), it establishes planning and participatory machinery. Offe argues, however, that the capitalist state is incapable of planning.

> Planning . . . seems to be inherently impossible in the capitalist state as an internal mode of operation—impossible not in itself, but because of the acts of retaliation that planning provokes on the part of capital as a whole or individual accumulating units. Such acts of retaliation (the major forms of which are *absolute* disinvestment, or investment strikes, and *relative* disinvestment, or displacement of investment in time and space) tend to make the cure worse than the disease under capitalism, and are thus self-paralyzing in regard to state activity.[25]

THE LIBERAL PERSPECTIVE

Liberals, like conservatives, also trace their beliefs to the British tradition of liberalism. Benjamin Ward summarizes the liberal theory of the nature of man in three concepts,

> hedonism, rationalism, and atomism. The first refers to the seeking of pleasure and the avoidance of pain, to human motivation as having a very strong materialistic, sensate side.

This side is sufficiently strong that it can be used as the basis for social analysis, though without losing sight of the nobler qualities that motivate humans from time to time.[26]

Although the underlying values of liberals resemble those of conservatives, there are some important differences. For example, personal responsibility for achievement is valued, but liberals do not insist that the link between rewards and effort should be maintained for all goods and services. They consider some goods and services as a right rather than a reward; thus, the concept of merit goods in public economics.

Freedom, too, is valued but there is also a broad role for state intervention. As Richard Tawney put it,

> There is no such thing as freedom in the abstract, divorced from the realities of a particuliar time and place. . . . It is still often assumed by privileged classes that, when the state refrains from intervening, the condition which remains, as a result of its inaction, is liberty. In reality, what not infrequently remains is not liberty, but tyranny. . . . The right to education is obviously impaired, if poverty arrests its use in mid-career; the right to the free choice of an occupation, if the expenses of entering a profession are prohibitive; the right to earn a living, if enforced unemployment is recurrent; the right to justice, if few men of small means can afford the cost of litigation.[27]

With regard to the theory of the modern state, post-World War II liberals depart significantly from conservatives for they identify with social democratic ideals and with the principles of the welfare state. Representative writings in this tradition range from those of John Kenneth Galbraith, Gunnar Myrdal, and Richard Titmuss to those of Robert Dahl, Charles Lindblom, Richard Musgrave, and Andrew Shonfield.[28]

Liberals tend to view the state as a mediating force that somehow aggregates individual preferences and pursues the public interest. In so doing, the state is presumed responsible for providing services to the population. For example, in his analysis of the role of the state in the economy, Musgrave distinguishes three branches of government: allocation, distribution, and stabilization. Within this scheme, there are three justifications for state intervention in the economy: (1) to correct market failures; (2) to redistribute income; and (3) to manipulate fiscal and monetary policies in order to affect aggregate demand. Within the liberal system of beliefs, as Walter Heller claimed in the sixties, the government can achieve "any combination of government services, income redistribution, and economic redistribution and economic stability we set our sights on."[29]

Another vision of the state within the liberal belief system is the organic one. Such a view is grounded in Rousseau's concept of the "general will," which is not necessarily equivalent to the will of all. Like the French notion of solidarity, the organic vision of the state can serve to unify a nation around the idea of mutual aid, national cooperation, and planning. As noted by Robert Alford and exemplified in Galbraith's work, the utopian image of the liberal perspective is the planned society.[30]

IMPLICATIONS FOR HEALTH PLANNING

Since the perspectives described above are broad orienting positions, the implications for health planning are not necessarily consistent with *all* of the beliefs. Nevertheless, the perspectives, as well as their implications, are significant for they command strong support and follow from a set of deeply held world views.

THE CONSERVATIVE PERSPECTIVE

Conservatives contend that state intervention in the organization of medical care should be strictly limited. They challenge health planning efforts insofar as they extend beyond such traditional issues of public health as immunization programs. The strength of the conservative critique lies partially in our ignorance. We do not know what constitutes a right distribution of health resources and there may, in fact, be no such concept since the choice involves a decision about what kind of distribution we desire rather than the solution of a technical problem. Planning requires some knowledge about what the future is likely to bring, some control over key actors in the health system, some agreed upon criteria to evaluate the current delivery system for medical care, and some capacity to monitor the system being planned.

Conservatives argue that these requirements are seriously deficient in the health sector. But even if they were not, health planning would most likely reduce the role of free markets in resource allocation and increase state intervention and administrative control.[31] Moreover, health planning is likely to diminish both professional autonomy and consumer choice. It is not surprising, therefore, that conservative analysts are among the leading critics of planning; they believe it cannot work. Instead of a planning system, they prefer that health policy promote either of two models of medical care organization: the professional or the free enterprise model.

THE PROFESSIONAL MODEL

The professional model of medical care organization is naturally advocated by professional medical associations such as the American Medical Association (AMA) in the United States and the Confédération des Syndicats Médicaux Français (CSMF) in France. It emphasizes the virtues of private medical practice on a fee-for-service basis—what the French call *la médecine libérale*. Professional medical associations have sedulously cultivated an image of private practice as a personal, symbiotic doctor-patient relationship. To defend their professionalism, they have appealed to the desirability of free market choice: selection of the physician by the patient, freedom of prescription by the doctor, professional confidentiality, and fee-for-service payment.

All aspects of the professional model have been systematically defended in a classic study by Mathew Lynch and Stanley Raphael. In answer to the question "Is there, then, any place for socialized medicine?" Lynch and Raphael conclude as follows:

> Since all experience shows and history attests to mankind's unquenchable thirst for freedom with justice, it follows that any system which limits freedom and justice, which imposes coercion and restricts voluntary effort toward self-betterment—has no place in the advanced and just society. A system which commits its citizens to mental and fiscal imprisonment, which in its aim to abolish uncertainties unavoidably eliminates opportunity and challenge, and leaves only the boredom of a limited certainty—such a system can only be regarded as *reactionary* in the historic evolutionary process of man.[32]

The essence of the professional model comes forth in clarion tones when Lynch and Raphael assert that the "basic doctor-patient relationship, which is the sine qua non of good medical care, is destroyed by all schemes that remove responsibility from the patient." They find further "attestation of the immutable nature of these truths" in the following citation from Plato:

> Athenian Stranger: And did you ever observe that there are two classes of patients in states, slaves and freemen; and the slave doctors run about and cure the slaves, or wait for them in the dispensaries—practitioners of this sort never talk to their patients individually, or let them talk about their own individual complaints? The slave doctor prescribes what mere experience suggests, as if he had exact knowledge; and when he has given his orders, like a tyrant, he rushes off with equal assurance to some other servant who is ill; and so he relieves the master of the house of the care of his invalid slaves. But the other doctor, who is a freeman, attends and practices upon freemen; and he carries his enquiries far back, and goes into the nature of the disorder; he enters into discourse with the patient and with his friends, and is at once getting information from the sick man, and also instructing him as far as he is able,

and he will not prescribe for him until he has first convinced
him; at last, when he has brought the patient more and more
under his persuasive influences and set him on the road to
health, he attempts to effect a cure. Now which is the better
way of proceeding in a physician?[33]

THE FREE ENTERPRISE MODEL

The free enterprise model of medical care organization is
advocated by certain economists, principally D. S. Lees and
Milton Friedman.[34] Like the proponents of the professional
model, Lees and Friedman value free market choice and
voluntary exchange. They differ from the former in that
the traditional doctor-patient relationship is not important
to them so long as new doctor-patient relationships allow
market choice. Lees contends that medical care differs little
in any of its characteristics from other goods and services
and consequently defends the position that competitive
markets in the health sector would produce an efficient
allocation of medical resources. Friedman agrees. Lees also
criticizes the monopoly of the medical profession over the
delivery of health care and challenges the notion that for
reasons of technical efficiency in production (maintenance
of standards), licensure is justified. Instead of licensure,
Friedman advocates a system of voluntary certification in
which anyone would be free to practice medicine "without
restriction except for legal and financial responsibility for
any harm done to others through fraud and negligence."[35]
    Relying largely on the work of Reuben Kessel, Friedman
criticizes the existence of price discrimination in medicine.[36]
His argument is that the power of trade unions, including
medical professional associations, restricts competition and
results in artificially high medical fees. Friedman argues
that the medical profession has preserved its monopoly
position by severely limiting entry into medical schools and
retarded technological development both in medicine and
in the organization of medical care. He interprets the

growth of the professions of osteopathy and chiropractic as a reaction to medical monopoly power and argues that such alternatives might well be of lower quality than medical practice would have been without entry restrictions. Finally, he likens the high quality medical care required under current licensure standards to Cadillac standards in the automobile industry. He argues that elimination of medical licensure would increase access and allocate medical resources more efficiently.

> Group practice in conjunction with hospitals would have grown enormously. Instead of individual practice plus large institutional hospitals conducted by governments or eleemosynary institutions, there might have developed medical partnerships or corporations—medical teams. . . . These medical teams—department stores of medicine, if you will—would be intermediaries between the patients and the physician. Being long-lived and immobile, they would have a great interest in establishing a reputation for reliability and quality. For the same reason, consumers would get to know their reputation. They would have the specialized skills to judge the quality of physicians; indeed, they would be the agent of the consumer in doing so, as the department store is now for many a product.[37]

THE RADICAL PERSPECTIVE

Like the conservatives, radicals also oppose state intervention in the health sector; but they do so for different reasons. There are two main radical perspectives on health care: those who favor socialized medicine and those who favor deprofessionalized medicine. Proponents of socialized medicine criticize state intervention, in general, and health planning, in particular, within the context of capitalism. They contend that the role of the state is constrained by pressures of private capital accumulation and that planning serves as a tool of monopoly capital.[38] Consequently, to achieve significant change, those who favor socialized medicine argue that one must first begin by changing the capitalist system. Proponents of deprofessionalized medicine criticize state intervention and planning because it expands bureaucratic control over the health sector. Consequently, they attack not merely capitalism but socialism as well; and they advocate debureaucratization.

SOCIALIZED MEDICINE

The case for socialized medicine grows out of a critique of private medical practice and a commitment to equity in the provision of medical care. Proponents of socialized medicine criticize the presence of the profit motive in the capitalist health sector.[39] They claim that even if most goods and services are distributed on the basis of the consumer's willingness to pay, this should not be the way medical care is distributed. Medical care is different.[40] It should be distributed on the basis of some principle of fairness. After all, we are all part of the human family and since a large part of illness falls on individuals because of fortuitous circumstances, they should not have to bear the costs alone. When health is threatened, since charity is insufficient to cope with our moral obligation to help those in need, the state must provide medical care to all. As Henry Sigerist put it many years ago,

> The goal of medicine is social. . . . Man has a right to health and is entitled to having this right secured . . . everybody, rich and poor, should have all the medical care that science can give. There is only one way of achieving this: the physician must be removed from the sphere of competitive business.[41]

In contrast to proponents of the professional model who claim that the doctor will look after the interest of the patient where there is a fee for services rendered, advocates of socialized medicine argue that the professional fee distorts the doctor-patient relationship. They contend that fee-for-service medicine tempts the doctor to pursue his own interests before those of the patients. As George Bernard Shaw put it,

> That any nation, having observed that you could provide for the supply of bread by giving bakers a pecuniary interest in baking for you, should go on to give a surgeon a pecuniary interest in cutting off your leg, is enough to make one despair of political humanity.[42]

Those who favor socialized medicine scoff at the notion that medical care should be bought and sold like a commodity.

> Under such a system, the sickest patient, whose needs are greatest, is at a disadvantage in this medical market, and his disadvantage is proportionate to his sickness. . . . The private practice of medicine is spotty and haphazard. It dictates the supply of physicians according to the harsh laws of economics and militates against the equitable distribution of physicians, so that the poor and those in depressed and rural areas—people whose needs are often the greatest—get the least medical care.[43]

A nationalized health service such as that in England (chaps. 4 and 7) involves public ownership of the hospital sector and allows a limited amount of private practice; but under socialized medicine such as in the Soviet model, private practice is prohibited by law, and *all* physicians work on a salaried basis for the state. In theory, such a model requires central planning and regionalization of health resources and is possible only in a socialist society.

DEPROFESSIONALIZED MEDICINE

The case for deprofessionalized medicine grows out of a critique of professionalism and bureaucracy in industrially advanced nations. Ivan Illich argues that damage done by medical providers—what he calls iatrogenesis—reflects the failure of our medical care system.[44] Illich advocates a total

debureaucratization of industrial society.[45] He delivers unsparing criticism at industrialism and claims that our medical delivery system has reached a point where advances in
medical technology result in an increasing incidence of
iatrogenesis:

> Medicine began to approach the second watershed. Every year
> medical science reported a new breakthrough. Practitioners of
> new specialties rehabilitated some individuals suffering from
> rare diseases. The practice of medicine became centered on
> the performance of hospital-based staffs. Trust in miracle
> cures obliterated good sense and traditional wisdom on heal-
> ing and health care. The irresponsible use of drugs spread
> from doctors to the general public. The second watershed was
> approached when the marginal utility of further professional-
> ization declined, at least insofar as it can be expressed in terms
> of the physical well-being of the largest numbers of people.
> The second watershed was superseded when the marginal
> *dis*utility increased as further monopoly of the medical estab-
> lishment became an indicator of more suffering for larger
> numbers of people.[46]

For Illich, there are three kinds of iatrogenesis: clinical,
social, and structural. Clinical iatrogenesis results from
pain, sickness, or death provoked by the provision of medical care. Social iatrogenesis results when health policies
reinforce an industrial organization that generates dependency and ill health. Structural iatrogenesis results when
"medically sponsored behavior and delusions restrict the
vital autonomy of people by undermining their competence
in growing up, caring for each other and aging."[47]

Illich proposes to limit the dependency that industrial
society imposes by fostering self-reliance, self-care, and consumer control over the provision of health services. This is
strangely reminiscent of Friedman's free enterprise model
of medical care organization. But it differs in that Illich is
not as concerned with free choice and pluralistic modes of
health care delivery as much as he is concerned with re-

ducing dependence on professional services and increasing individual autonomy and self-sufficiency.

THE LIBERAL PERSPECTIVE

In contrast to conservatives and radicals, liberals support both state intervention in the health sector, in general, and health planning, in particular. Liberals do not seek fundamental changes in the present role of the modern welfare state. They accept the present institutional arrangements for financing and organizing health care; consequently, they focus their attention on pragmatic state intervention to minimize current problems. Although there are no clearly articulated models of how a liberal health sector in the United States would look, liberals would most likely support a national health insurance program to improve access to health services and a range of administrative controls and financial incentives to contain rising health care costs.

Liberals occupy a midway position between conservatives and radicals. They support aspects of the conservative's professional and free-enterprise models of medical care organization; at the same time they are sympathetic to aspects of socialized and deprofessionalized medicine. For example, along with advocates of the professional model, liberals support the enforcement of minimal licensing standards for health professionals and hospitals. Along with advocates of the free-enterprise model, they favor the use of market incentives to improve efficiency in the allocation of health resources. In addition, liberals share the equity concerns of advocates of socialized medicine and they support the concerns about self-reliance and consumer control expressed by advocates of deprofessionalization.

Dispute among liberals and conservatives about the proper role of the state in the health sector usually centers on the following questions: how extensive is market failure in health care? How great is the inability of the market to satisfy the rights of individuals to medical care? At one extreme, left-leaning liberals advocate a state controlled national health service along the lines of the English model. At the other extreme, right-leaning conservatives advocate private health insurance allocated on the basis of ability to pay market premiums.

Economists have noted the special characteristics of medical care which make it an unattractive candidate for efficient allocation by the market mechanism.[48] To view the matter only from the economic perspective, however, does not provide a satisfactory basis for evaluating the proper role of the market versus the state in the organization of medical care. Economist Anthony Culyer put it this way:

> nothing scientific can (at the moment) be said about the relative desirability of the NHS (or any other system) and consequently . . . social scientists (or any other kind) who believe that they have shown that general circumstances can determine the best form of organization of medical care, are in fact, wittingly or unwittingly, lending spurious support to what amounts to no more than an ideological assertion.[49]

Liberals and conservatives do not disagree about the existence of market failure in the health sector. Rather, they have different criteria for evaluating the appropriateness of state intervention and planning. The liberal perspective is characterized by three central criteria that should guide state intervention in the health sector: rationality, equity, and accountability.

RATIONALITY

Max Weber distinguished between two kinds of rationality: substantive rationality, which refers to the value of desired goals; and formal rationality, which refers to the effectiveness of particular means used to advance any specified end.[50] Liberals concentrate on the latter category: the relation between means and ends. In the spirit of British economic liberalism, conservatives argue that formally rational behavior of individuals pursuing their own self-interest tends to promote a notion of public interest that is substantively rational. In contrast, liberals note that a society whose members act in a formally rational way, or even one whose members are individually substantively rational, is not necessarily a rational society in the sense of successfully achieving its shared values. Along with Weber, liberals would interpret state intervention and planning as attempts to harness the market for purposes of improving economic efficiency and achieving a "rational society."

Planners tend to adopt a cognitive style of defining goals, assessing alternative strategies to achieve them, and evaluating the impact of these strategies. For example, health planners have emphasized a broad definition of health (see Appendix 1, fig. 15), evaluated the effectiveness of medical care, and urged more comprehensive health interventions on forces outside the medical sector. To the extent that they have set priorities, analyzed perceived problems, and evaluated alternatives and results, they may be said to be acting rationally. In this sense, liberals have embraced a renewed faith in state intervention and comprehensive planning to rationalize the health sector.

EQUITY

In addition to their concern for formal rationality, liberals appeal to ideals about what a good health system should do. They tend to use the notion of equity to encompass a range of these ideals. Social, political, and moral theorists, for example, appeal to the notion of rights as well as to justice and fairness.[51] Often these criteria have been used to justify the redistribution of health resources away from groups who have plenty to those who are in need, such as between relatively underserved and overserved regions of the country or between the poor and the affluent. In this sense, it is important to distinguish equity from equality. Whereas equality of medical care implies an equal amount for all, equity implies a distribution based on such principles as "To each his due" or "To him that hath, from him, much shall be required,"[52] that is to say, care in accordance with some criteria of "need," not ability to purchase.

The equity criterion can be used to justify state intervention even when the market results in an efficient allocation of resources, for such a result is not necessarily equitable. To the extent that liberal theorists rely on equity as a criterion for state intervention when the market would otherwise operate efficiently, they agree with radicals. But when there is evidence of market failure, then the liberal's appeal to equity is strengthened. In the absence of the free market's obtaining an efficient allocation, an even stronger case can be made for the pursuit of justice.

ACCOUNTABILITY

Often, the pursuit of equity has led liberals to advocate greater centralization of planning such as the elaboration of national standards for the allocation of new medical technology. Centralization, however, conflicts with goals of local autonomy and raises the issue of accountability.

The market distributes resources in response to impersonal forces; politics is responsive to interest groups, institutions and corporations, which have power. Thus, liberals advocate the design of institutional mechanisms to hold health care providers and planners accountable and responsive to key actors in the health sector. The challenge in making these ideals operational lies in defining the relevant groups, which, among others, may include residents of a region, subscribers to insurance, health care workers, consumers, or some combination of these.

IMPLICATIONS FOR THIS STUDY

The basic differences in perspectives on the state cannot be resolved—or ignored—in this study. I will return to them in chapter 9 because these broad perspectives on the proper role of the state in society inspire alternative explanations as to why implementation of health planning is so difficult to achieve.

The conservative perspective supports the view that regulatory strategies will not succeed in rationalizing the health sector. Analysts of this persuasion might emphasize the limited applicability of modern management methods to problems in the health sector. The radical perspective focuses on the inability of the state to pursue planning within the capitalist system. These analysts emphasize the systemic constraints to state intervention in the health sector such as requirements of capital accumulation.

Only the liberal perspective accepts the legitimacy and ability of the state to solve social problems within modern capitalism. But even this perspective calls attention to the formidable obstacles to social reform. Analysts in this tradition note the resistance by "structural interests," which produces stalemate in health care politics.

Conservative, radical, and liberal perspectives on the state suggest different grounds for evaluating alternative modes of state intervention. But they do not yield specific prescriptions about the kind of planning that ought to be promoted in the health sector. To get at these issues I will distinguish six kinds of health planning in the case studies and evaluate how each has functioned in different contexts and at different stages of health sector development. In the next chapter, I will analyze how health planning goals could be implemented, in theory, primarily from a liberal perspective, but keeping in mind the criticisms of conservatives and radicals.

3

HEALTH PLANNING
AND IMPLEMENTATION

Before examining what health planners have actually done in practice, it is useful to review some of the difficulties they confront and how, in theory, these difficulties might be overcome. This chapter begins by considering two aspects of the health planning predicament: how to set standards for the proper allocation of health resources and how to secure implementation of health plans. Next, it analyzes the behavior of consumers and providers of medical care and examines a range of policy instruments to implement health planning goals. The use of such instruments appears likely to be effective only to the extent that policymakers link health planning activities to the institutions involved in health care financing: third party payers, rate setters, and budgetary authorities. Thus, the final section of this chapter makes a case for linking health planning and financing. To forge effective linkages, the social goals of reimbursement must coincide with those of health planning. The following analysis, however, suggests that it is no easy task to devise operational criteria that serve this end.

THE HEALTH PLANNING PREDICAMENT

Although there is general agreement among policymakers that all people should have access to medical care regardless of income or place of residence, health planners are unable to specify what constitutes an optimal system of health and social services for keeping a target population healthy. They resort to stating—sometimes with great eloquence—the current opinion about what constitutes an improved health system. There is a consensus for the necessity of challenging the predominant medical model of hospital-centered care and promoting redistribution of health resources from hospitals to public health services and community-based health and social services. But even with a consensus, health planners most often fail to carry out the plans they formulate. In short, the predicament of health planning is that no one knows how to assure that the right patient receives the right service at the right time and in the right place; and even when a consensus is reached on what is "right," critical elements of plans, policies, and programs are rarely implemented.

THE PROBLEM OF STANDARDS

A look at the health planning literature suggests that neither planners nor physicians know how much medical care is "needed" for particular populations, how much is lacking, or what is the best way of providing medical services.[1] What we know, on the basis of cross-national comparisons, is that different nations have organized their health services according to divergent conceptions of what is "right." The level of health resources and the standards of medical care differ greatly around the world. Whether one looks at health expenditures as a percent of GDP (gross domestic product), or at the number of physicians and hospital beds per capita, there is considerable variation among nations (table 2).[2] For example, among industrially advanced nations, the relationship between lengths of stay and admission rates in hospitals reveals that nations of geographic proximity have similar patterns of hospital utilization (fig. 3). Overall, however, the amount of variation is tremendous.

TABLE 2
Variation in Actual Health Resources

Country	Health expenditures as percentage of GDP		General hospital beds per 10,000 population 1971	Physicians per 10,000 population 1971	Nurses per 10,000 population 1970
	Year	Percentage	Number	Number	Number
North America					
Canada	1973	6.8	54.7[2]	15.1	45.9
United States	1974	7.4	46.7	15.4	35.3
Great Britain					
England and Wales	1975	5.2[1]	40.7	12.7	30.7
Scotland	—	—	49.4	15.6	35.5
Scandinavia					
Sweden	1974	7.3	69.4	13.9	40.7
Western Group					
The Netherlands	1972	7.3	53.6	13.2	19.2
Belgium	1974	5.0	47.3[2]	16.0[3]	— —
Luxembourg	1974	4.0	58.9	10.8	19.6
France	1974	6.9	60.5	13.9	26.6
Southern Group					
Italy	1974	6.0	48.3	18.4[3]	6.9
Spain	1974	4.8	31.3	13.9[4]	6.7
Portugal	—	—	37.9	9.7	4.5
Central Group					
West Germany	1968	6.1	66.8	17.8	23.1
Austria	1968	5.6	60.1[2]	18.7[3]	20.3
Switzerland	1965	3.8	60.3	15.0	22.8

Source: Data on health expenditures are from *Public Expenditure on Health* (Paris: OECD Studies in Resource Allocation, 1977). Data on hospital beds, physicians, and nurses are from R. Maxwell, *Health Care: The Growing Dilemma. Needs v. Resources in Western Europe, the U. S. and the U. S. S. R.* 2d ed. (New York: McKinsey, 1975), pp. 69–71.

[1] This figure is for the United Kingdom.
[2] For 1970.
[3] Includes those practicing dentistry.
[4] Registered personnel only.

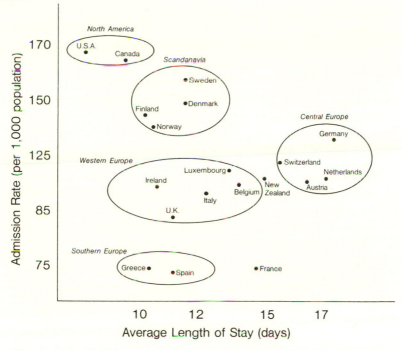

Fig. 3. Hospital lengths of stay and admission rates in different nations.

*The data are from *World Statistics Annuals* (Geneva: WHO, 1973).

Source: J. F. Lacronique, "Cross-Sectional International Analysis of the Consumption of Short-Term Hospital Care," masters thesis (Sloan School of Management, Massachusetts Institute of Technology, June 1977), p. 34.

There are also significant disparities in professionally set standards for medical care. For example, standards for the allocation of specialized medical equipment such as CT scanners (computerized axial tomography) range from one per 100,000 population in the United States to one per 2 million population in Great Britain (table 3). Despite their apparently arbitrary nature, standards within particular nations serve as convenient rules by which to allocate scarce resources equitably.[3] In the absence of agreement on technical solutions to the issue of how much medical care is needed, the dominant professional groups have, so far, controlled the process of standard setting. But as the process of health planning includes broader participation, planners are likely to replace professional standards with more broadly consensual processes for deciding what constitutes a proper distribution of health resources.

According to our definition, reaching a consensus on what is right is only part of the health planning predicament. Nathan Glazer notes that

> if the limitations on our knowledge were the only problem in the way of effective health planning, all health planners would rejoice, for these technical and scientific difficulties and complexities in the way of the provision of good medical care pale when we consider the political and economic difficulties.[4]

Glazer is referring to the other dimension of the health planning predicament: implementing health plans—transforming policy into practice.[5]

The Problem of Implementation

Studies of implementation tend to focus only on part of the problem, and the easy part at that. In a review of the literature, Eugene Bardach discerns five major themes: pressure politics, the massing of "assent," administrative control, intergovernmental bargaining, and the complexity of joint action.[6]

Scholars writing about implementation focus on "what happens after a bill becomes a law" or "how policies change as they are translated from administrative guidelines into practice."[7] They have produced incisive analyses of the vast number of interest groups affected by particular government policies, the multiple levels of decision making, and the complexity of "getting things done." But by focusing on the organizational issues of decision making these studies tend to suffer from "misplaced concreteness." For example, in their book, *Implementation*, Pressman and Wildavsky enumerate thirty "decision points" in the course of imple-

TABLE 3
STANDARDS FOR CT SCANNERS* IN 1978

	Population per CT scanner
United States[1]	
Indiana	100,000
Colorado	225,000[2]
Alabama	500,000[2]
Netherlands	450,000
Japan	500,000
Canada	1,000,000
France	1,000,000
Great Britain	2,000,000

Sources: Indiana: D. Banta, ed., *Policy Implications of the Computed Tomography (CT) Scanner* (Washington, D.C.: Office of Technology Assessment, August 1978), p. 59; Colorado and Indiana: *A Health Planning Document: Computerized Tomographic Scanning Systems* (Cambridge, Mass.: Arthur D. Little, prepared under contract with the Health Resources Administration, U. S. DHEW, November 1976), p. 75; figures for other countries are cited by J. de Kervasdoué, "Les politiques de santé sont-elles adaptées à la pratique de la médecine?" *Sociologie du Travail* 3 (1979).
*Includes head and body scanners.
[1] In the United States, there was never a population-based federal standard for CT scanners. The 1978 National Health Planning Guidelines (Federal Register, Washington, D.C., March 28, 1978) recommended that a CT scanner "should operate at a minimum of 2,500 medically necessary patient procedures per year, for the second year of its operation and thereafter."
[2] These figures are for 1975–1976.

menting the Economic Development Administration's Oakland projects. They foresaw seventy necessary "agreements" and a .000395 probability of program success, assuming that the probability of each agreement was as high as .95.[8]

Bardach well reflects the characteristic tone of the literature on implementation when he laments,

It is hard enough to design public policies and programs that look good on paper. It is harder still to formulate them in words and slogans that resonate pleasingly in the ears of political leaders and the constituencies to which they are responsive. And it is excruciatingly hard to implement them in a way that pleases anyone at all including the supposed beneficiaries or clients.[9]

He concludes his book, *The Implementation Game*, by urging that we become "more modest in our demands on, and expectations of, the institutions of representative government."[10]

Whether our "demands on and expectations of" government should become more modest is a moot question. What seems more certain is that in the modern welfare state it is practically impossible to separate those who pay from those who receive disproportionate benefits from government. Hugh Heclo notes,

> The difference in degree of dependence is hardly self-evident between a single mother receiving public assistance, free medical care and welfare milk, and the rugged individualist dependent only on the tax law for subsidizing interest payments on his otherwise too-costly home, state enforced credit regulations to multiply his purchasing power, tax indulgences for his lucrative retirement plan and expense account, and government agencies planning to make others bear the social costs of urban renewal, private transportation and fighting inflation.[11]

Given the all-pervasive nature of government in industrially advanced nations, the intellectually interesting question, and also the relevant one for policy, is not whether there should be more or less government but rather whose interests should be served and how to affect resource allocation accordingly.

Most of the literature on implementation reflects a bias toward the conservative perspective on the proper role of the state in society. It tends to emphasize organizational politics and the more general quandaries of decision making. But such an approach diverts attention from dominant producer groups such as the medical profession, which shape legislation in the first place and prevent it from meeting its proclaimed objectives when the legislation is not in their interests. By focusing on the decision as its unit of analysis, scholars writing about implementation divert attention from more structural issues.

Every system has certain built-in biases in favor of one sort of behavior rather than another.[12] In the health sector, the structure of financial incentives could encourage hospital-centered care or public health services, preventive medicine, and social services. More often than not, it favors the former. Thus, the more intractable dimension of the implementation problem is how to change the incentives of the health system.

MEDICAL CARE SYSTEM BEHAVIOR AND THE OPTIONS FOR PLANNED INTERVENTION

Although there is no general theory of health systems, we can posit some modest claims about the behavior of medical care providers and consumers, and about the impact of alternative financial incentives on them.[13] To begin with, let us consider five propositions about the nature of the medical care system and explore their implications. This exercise should shed some light on the ways in which health planners can affect the behavior of hospitals and physicians; and consequently on how they might achieve greater control over the allocation of health resources.

PROPOSITIONS

1. There are no clear limits on what a medical care system can or should spend.

This proposition derives from two principles that appear to operate in the world of medicine for the bulk of the population able to voice their views. First is the technological imperative. As Jacques Ellul observes, "that which is technologically possible appears necessary to public opinion . . . and public opinion would not tolerate the failure to realize what is possible."[14] Second, there is always something else that can be done in medicine—another consultation, a different drug, an alternative therapy. Wildavsky calls this the "medical uncertainty principle."[15]

2. Since the consumer is a poor judge of both the effec-
    tiveness and the efficiency of medical care, he gen-
    erally relies on the physician as his agent in deter-
    mining the type and quantity of services demanded.
    The traditional free market model of a "sovereign
    consumer" does not hold in the health sector. In-
    formation costs are high, illness is generally involun-
    tary and unpredictable, and there are many con-
    straints on the availability of alternative sources of
    care.

3. Health insurance coverage by third-party payers
    eliminates most of the financial burden on consumers
    and allows providers almost open-ended financing.
    Physicians are generally reimbursed on the basis
    of "usual, customary, and reasonable" (UCR) fees.
    Hospitals are generally reimbursed on the basis of
    costs incurred. And quality control mechanisms, such
    as Physician Standard Review Organizations (PSROs),
    have not significantly affected the aggregate volume
    of medical services produced.[16]

4. Provider reimbursement incentives are powerfully
    skewed toward specialized, high-cost care.[17]
    Professional prestige pushes physicians to special-
    ize. In addition, future income expectations and re-
    imbursement incentives encourage specialty medical
    care. Finally, fee-for-service payment rewards the
    multiplication of services and the provision of expen-
    sive care.

5. The medical care system has no ongoing mechanism
    to monitor systematically the outcomes of medical
    treatment, nor is any provider accountable for the
    patient's health beyond the services that he or she
    renders. (The risk of malpractice litigation tends to
    make physicians responsible only for the services they
    render.)

As Alberta Parker has noted with respect to primary health care services, "responsibility is unassigned and, therefore, unassumed."[18] Physicians and hospitals are only responsible for the medical services they provide, not for the final product of their services—individual health—and emphatically not for the health of a designated population at risk.

IMPLICATIONS

All five propositions imply that the medical care system will be characterized by the generous provision of technically sophisticated medical procedures and subject to strong physician-induced cost escalation. From propositions 1 (no limits) and 2 (physician as agent), it follows that providers have considerable latitude in determining the type and use of medical services that local populations will receive. From proposition 3 (health insurance coverage), it follows that physicians will tend to locate where they find it most congenial. And from proposition 4 (provider reimbursement incentives), it follows that physicians will tend to specialize. Finally, proposition 5 (no monitoring of outcomes) suggests that the medical care system will tend to emphasize the provision of medical services and to neglect the relative importance of other "inputs to health" (see fig. 15 in Appendix 1). All these inferences are supported by empirical findings.

In addition, all five propositions have implications for health planning. In particular, those concerning health insurance coverage, provider reimbursement incentives, and monitoring of outcomes (3, 4, and 5), involve behavioral characteristics of medical care systems that can be affected by public policy. Thus, health planners can attempt to alter the conditions on which the propositions are based. Proposition 5 refers to medical care organization, and propositions 3 and 4 refer to financial incentives for consumers and providers. These are interrelated; for the range of financial incentives is limited by the context of medical care organization, while such changes in health care financing as the passage of national health insurance can be used as leverage to effect organizational change.[19] With regard to implementation, it is critical for health planners to understand the impact of financial incentives on the behavior of both providers and consumers of medical care.

THE IMPACT OF FINANCIAL INCENTIVES

A wide variety of institutional arrangements now govern the delivery of medical care; but, for purposes of analysis, we will distinguish six distinct types (table 4).[20] These arrangements can affect aggregate health care costs and the distribution of health resources.

The columns and rows in table 4 represent the direct marginal financial impact on consumers and providers each

TABLE 4

IMPACT OF FINANCIAL INCENTIVES ON MEDICAL CARE PROVIDERS AND CONSUMERS

Marginal financial impact on provider each time a service is rendered	Marginal financial impact on consumer each time a service is received	
	A. Negative	B. Zero
C. Positive	CA (Fee-for-service without insurance or high coinsurance)	CB (First-dollar insurance coverage with fee-for-service reimbursement)
B. Zero	BA (An outpatient department in a hospital charging patients a fee)	BB (A national health service as, for example, in England)
A. Negative	AA (Prepayment with some utilization fees)	AB (Prepayment without utilization fees—HMOs)

Source: Adapted from table 1 in U. Reinhardt, "Alternative Methods of Reimbursing Non-Institutional Providers of Health Services," *Controls on Health Care*, Papers of the Conference on Regulation in the Health Industry, January 7–9, 1974 (Washington, D.C.: Institute of Medicine, National Academy of Sciences, 1975), p. 141.

time a medical service is received or rendered. On the consumer side, column A refers to medical systems either without any health insurance coverage or with a combination of insurance and high coinsurance and deductibles (i.e., out-of-pocket payments by consumers). Column B refers to medical systems where medical care is free at the point of consumption—either a national health insurance (NHI) system, a national health service (NHS), or a prepayment system, such as a health maintenance organization (HMO) in the United States. On the provider side, row C refers to traditional fee-for-service reimbursement. Row B refers to a system where economic returns are invariant with respect to the amount of services provided—for example, full average cost reimbursement for hospitals and salary payment for physicians. And row A refers to a system under which providers deliver medical care against some form of prepayment and face incentives to minimize utilization.

Given assumptions 2 (the physician as agent) and 3 (health insurance coverage), whatever the price elasticity of demand for medical services, consumers facing zero prices (cells CB, BB, and AB) will tend, other things being equal, to utilize more medical services than consumers facing out-of-pocket payments (cells CA, BA, or AA). Shonick and Roemer present such evidence in the case of HMOs;[21] Bunker provides further evidence in his study of surgical interventions in England and the United States;[22] and empirical economic studies demonstrate that reimbursement incentives affect physician behavior at the margin.[23]

In addition to affecting medical care utilization, provider reimbursement mechanisms affect efficiency in the production of medical services. There are no conclusive studies on the relative efficiency in the provision of physician services between health systems where the marginal financial impact on the physician is negative as opposed to positive (rows A and C). Nor is there conclusive evidence about hospital efficiency between rows A and C. With regard to hospitals, economists are increasingly critical of the traditional open-ended mode of retrospective reimbursement on the basis of costs incurred.[24] There have been a number of experiments involving prospective reimbursement of hospitals, where daily rates are established in advance and hospitals are paid regulated rates regardless of the costs actually incurred. There have also been experiments with systems of budget review. But the results are not yet decisive.[25]

Finally, provider reimbursement mechanisms could even affect the geographic and specialty distribution of physicians. Although the literature on the determinants of physician location indicates that financial incentives play a minor role in the physician's locational choice,[26] the present structure of reimbursement incentives under Medicare and Medicaid appears to reinforce the uneven distribution of specialist physicians. As shown in table 5, prevailing Medicare charges of specialists in 1975 were an average of 33 percent higher in counties with more than 175 physi-

TABLE 5

MEAN AND RANGE FOR MEDICARE AND MEDICAID SPECIALIST FEE INDICES
BY
COUNTY PHYSICIAN-POPULATION RATIO, 1975

	Number of counties	Medicare		Medicaid	
		Mean	Range	Mean	Range
All counties	3,074	100	70–192	100	49–179
Physicians per 100,000 population (1973)					
24	314	85	71–126	108	61–145
25–74	1,747	85	70–126	101	49–154
75–124	704	82	70–132	99	49–179
125–174	182	102	71–154	103	49–142
175–224	70	113	75–154	102	49–150
225–299	25	110	77–154	94	49–134
300+	32	113	80–192	90	49–145

Source: "Physician Payment Incentives," *Health Care Financing Review* (Summer 1979), p. 75; Medicare Carrier Survey, Intermediary Letter 74-19 (June 1974); Medicaid State Survey, SRS Action Transmittal 75-25 (June 1975).

cians per 100,000 population than in counties with fewer than 75 physicians per 100,000 population. As to specialty distribution, practitioner/specialist reimbursement differentials and slower rates of growth in allowed charges for primary care specialties suggest that the Medicare program provides no financial incentives for physicians to choose primary-care specialties.[27]

POLICY INSTRUMENTS AND TARGETS

From the experience of Western industrial nations, one can distinguish a broad range of policy instruments that the central government has at its disposal. These are summarized in table 6.[28] The assumption is that it might be possible to direct these instruments at specific targets and, thus, bring an actual situation closer to the desired one.

At the risk of drastic oversimplification, table 6 distinguishes four principal targets and three categories of policy instruments. Within the health sector, the state may direct its policy instruments to influence both the demand and the supply of health services. On the demand side, the state may seek to affect the behavior of all consumers or attempt to discriminate among potential consumers—the covered population or subscribers—and actual users of services. For example, the state may pass a health insurance program and design eligibility criteria (administrative incentives), impose cost-sharing provisions (market incentives), and promote antismoking campaigns (moral incentives). On the supply side, the state may seek to affect the behavior of providers—hospitals and physicians. For example, it may legislate hospital subsidy programs and regulate hospital expansion (administrative incentives), design market incentives for reimbursing physicians and hospitals, and encourage changes in medical ethics (moral incentives), such as legitimating euthanasia under certain conditions.

Outside of the health sector, the state may direct its policy instruments to subnational units of administration. This is

TABLE 6
POLICY INSTRUMENTS AND TARGETS IN THE HEALTH SECTOR

Targets	Administrative incentives	*Instruments* Market incentives	Moral incentives
Consumers: Subscribers Users	eligibility rules for health insurance	complementary insurance coverage cost-sharing (out-of-pocket payments)	health education programs health promotion campaigns
Providers: Hospitals Physicians	global budgeting limits on capital investment licensing standards utilization review peer review fees schedules	prospective reimbursement tax deductions subsidies advertising reduction in entry barriers	medical ethics
Administration: Ministries Subnational units	standards program planning evaluation	matching funds	demonstration projects social experiments
Firms	standards for health and safety standards for quality of drugs or food products	tax deductions (for health insurance premiums) merit rating in determination of health insurance premiums	preventive programs, e.g. screening

particularly important in federal systems such as the United States and Canada where the federal government may provide irresistible incentives for state and provincial levels to enact specified programs—for example, Medicaid in the United States and national health insurance in Canada. The federal government can also provide matching funds as well as leadership and exhortation (moral incentives) for subnational administrative units to set up demonstration projects or even social experiments. In addition to influencing subnational administrative units, the state may seek to influence the behavior of firms. For example, it may require them to establish occupational health and safety programs and to provide comprehensive health benefits to their employees. It may also impose specified safety regulations and create fiscal incentives for the provision of comprehensive health benefits to their employees.

Looking across the columns of table 6, one sees that the three categories of policy instruments cover a wide range of mechanisms for state intervention in the health sector. To some extent, the state may enact policies that rely on the use of administrative incentives as well as on the use of market and moral incentives. In addition, it may implement such legislation through the judicious use of administrative, market, and moral incentives. In this sense, there is overlap between categories of policy instruments. But such overlap does not change the fact that health planners usually rely on some combination of these mechanisms to implement explicit policy goals.

Health planning activities generally precede and follow the use of all policy instruments noted in table 6. For example, health planners design and evaluate the effects of administrative, market, and moral incentives. As state intervention in the health sector has increased, the range and number of policy instruments and targets have increased, as well. The optimal mix of policy instruments is presumably one that would induce the critical actors in the health sector (targets) to behave in accordance with explicitly agreed-upon social goals. In practice, social goals are most often vague, numerous, and conflicting, and there is no theory that specifies the optimal mix of policy instruments for achieving given social goals. The mechanisms of state intervention and, indeed, even the decision to intervene are most frequently based on ideological predispositions about the proper role of the state in society (chap. 2).

Some analysts holding conservative beliefs emphasize the importance of recreating the market in the health sector. With regard to firms, a number of ideas can be devised within such a framework. For example, merit rating on the basis of occupational hazards at the workplace could be used in the determination of employer health insurance premiums. For consumers, cost sharing is emphasized and, for providers, emphasis is placed on dismantling the regulatory system and encouraging advertising and market competition.

Other analysts holding liberal beliefs reject these notions as romantic and put the burden back on regulatory strategies.[29] They advocate the judicious use of government policy instruments that take into account the behavior of the medical care system. For example, in the United States, they would advocate the use of such administrative incentives as a national fee schedule for physicians, prospective reimbursement for hospitals and quality controls on patterns of medical practice.

THE NEED FOR AND THE PROBLEMS OF LINKING
HEALTH PLANNING AND FINANCING

Among health planners in the United States, there is currently a consensus that reimbursement incentives have, as yet, failed to promote health planning goals. They have failed, in particular, to contain health care costs and to substitute community-based health and social services for hospital-based institutional care. Such a view postulates that the critical policy targets are hospitals and physicians and that the critical combination of policy instruments are administrative and market incentives. Indeed, to implement health planning goals, there is a need to improve links between health planning activities and those institutions responsible for financing health care. Such institutions include all third party payers, public authorities charged with the regulation of provider reimbursement rates, and government agencies that determine budgets for hospitals and public health programs.

Karen Davis, a former assistant secretary for Planning and Evaluation in the Department of Health and Human Services, has recommended aggressive use of reimbursement incentives to discourage costly institutional care and to encourage primary health services.[30] She advocates: (1) reduction of physician fees for institutional services; (2) elimination of financial incentives to prescribe costly medical procedures; (3) relatively higher payments for primary health services, particularly in rural areas; (4) a means of reimbursement that favors comprehensive and primary health centers; (5) salary reimbursement of hospital-based physicians; and (6) continued experimentation with new methods of hospital reimbursement, for example, prospective budgeting.

With regard to hospitals, Katherine Bauer, who directed the most thorough studies on the theme of linkage, states the case succinctly:

> Rate-setting is now being looked to as a possible means of putting teeth into the future reviews of existing institutional services, through application of reimbursement penalties on institutions whose services are found to be inappropriate.[31]

There is little disagreement among health planners about the desirability of using reimbursement incentives to promote health planning goals. There are problems, however, in resolving the practical issues of how linkage can be achieved and in choosing appropriate criteria to make it operational and subsequently evaluate the effects of alternative reimbursement mechanisms.

To link health planning and financing, the social goals of reimbursement must correspond to those of health planning. Ideally, the reimbursement system should encourage physicians and hospitals to provide services based more on medical reasons than on financial incentives at the margin. This goal raises the question of what criteria to use in evaluating the effects of alternative reimbursement mechanisms.

For evaluating the effects of alternative methods of physician reimbursement, William Glaser suggests the following criteria: encouragement of good medicine, prevention of abuse, discouragement of neglect, and recruitment and allocation of doctors.[32] Although these criteria reflect important social goals, they need to be made more operational. How, for example, is one to measure good medicine and specify what constitutes a proper distribution of physicians? What is a reasonable rate of return to physicians? Is it possible to manage physician-induced demand? In designing payment mechanisms that link health planning to physician reimbursement, planners cannot escape such issues.

For evaluating the effects of alternative hospital reimbursement mechanisms, Paul Feldstein suggests the following criteria: internal hospital efficiency, efficiency in the allocation of resources among hospitals, control of increases in hospital expenditures, and minimization of the costs of medical treatment.[33] All these go well beyond current cost-based reimbursement practices, which derive their notions of "fairness" and "reasonableness" of payment from ways of assuring an acceptable flow of revenues over expenditures. Such criteria, however, do not provide guidelines for broader planning issues: To what extent, for example, should hospital reimbursement be the primary source of capital funds? Which regions require disproportionate investment and improved access to hospital and other health services? Further, these criteria are not helpful in specifying how to build incentives into the reimbursement scheme. Should reimbursement rates apply to medical procedures, hospital days or, more broadly, to illness episodes or the characteristics of the subscriber population?

Deriving criteria to evaluate alternatives in provider reimbursement ultimately forces recognition of a critical planning dilemma: how to create a reimbursement system in the health sector that encourages hospitals and physicians to pursue the interests of society as well as their own. This dilemma is yet another formulation of the health planning predicament.

The problem of implementing health planning goals involves no less than squaring the circle of private and public interests. Analyses of implementation and of medical care system behavior are helpful insofar as they point to the importance of linking health planning and financing. But practical issues of how to achieve linkage and what problems to anticipate are better understood by examining the experience of health planning in different institutional environments.

PART III
CASE STUDIES

4

PROFILES OF HEALTH SYSTEMS

As a preface to the case studies of health planning efforts, this chapter provides profiles of the health systems in the United States, France, the Canadian province of Québec, and England. It highlights the broad institutional structure of these health systems, the financing and organization of medical care, and the principal mechanisms of provider reimbursement.

HEALTH SYSTEMS COMPARED: AN OVERVIEW

THE UNITED STATES

The health system in the United States is characterized by its diversity, its pluralism, its emphasis on a large role for the private sector, and its cooperative federalism which justifies an active role for government intervention in promoting the general welfare.[1] The United States has no universal and compulsory national health insurance (NHI) program but it does provide public financing for the elderly and the very poor. The structure of the health system reflects a century of social reform that has been guided by three principles: liberalism, accountability, and equity. *Liberalism* refers to the nineteenth-century European sense of laissez-faire, individualism, and free choice. In the health sector, it implies the selection of the physician by the patient and vice

versa, freedom of prescription by the doctor, and professional confidentiality. *Accountability* refers to the notion
that professionals as well as public officials are ultimately
responsible to the people they serve. *Equity* appeals to a
notion of justice and provides the rationale for redistribution through government intervention.

Since these principles are not necessarily consistent with
one another, the structure of the health sector in the United
States reflects the impact of often contradictory policies.
Under the banner of liberalism and accountability the federal government has restricted its activities in the health
sector to encouraging pluralism and decentralization.
Under the banner of equity, and more recently "cost control," the federal government has pursued a policy of pragmatic state intervention.

Beginning in 1912, American reformers initiated a campaign to establish a system of universal and compulsory
NHI. At each stage of this campaign, however, efforts at
overall reform were defeated. In the course of successive
defeats, the policy agenda changed and other incremental
reforms were undertaken. There were grants to states for
the development of public health programs, for example,
maternal and child health services. In addition, there were
subsidies for the development of health resources (hospitals, biomedical research, and manpower), tax exemptions
for private health insurance premiums, health insurance
programs for the elderly and the very poor, and a maze of
categorical health programs for particular groups within
the population, for example, migrant workers.

In the 1930s, following the Great Depression, hospitals
coopted the efforts of American reformers to pass NHI
legislation and organized a system of private hospital insurance—Blue Cross. The insurance was designed as much to
benefit hospitals as it was to protect those who might need
hospital care. Following World War II, a period of rapid
health sector expansion began. In 1946 the Hill-Burton Act

provided federal subsidies for hospital construction and modernization. These subsidies increased throughout the 1950s and 1960s and were extended to encourage the growth of rural health facilities and nursing homes. Although the federal government pursued no explicit policies to increase the level of public financing, its implicit policies, such as allowing tax exemptions on the health insurance premiums purchased by employers for their employees, encouraged the rapid growth of private health insurance. In addition, federal support for biomedical research and training grew rapidly and began to transform the nation's medical schools, particularly those that were part of the major universities.

In the sixties, during the "war on poverty," the federal government actively intervened to improve access to health services. In 1965 a program of health insurance for the elderly (Medicare) and the poor (Medicaid) was finally passed. A network of regional medical programs was also established to narrow the gap between new biomedical knowledge and its application in specialized teaching hospitals. In addition, the Comprehensive Health Planning Act required states and local communities to set up planning agencies to identify health needs and strategies for meeting them. Finally, a variety of categorical programs was funded to provide health services to particular target populations— for example, neighborhood health centers (NHCs) for the poor, primary health care programs for migrant workers, maternal and infant care projects, and new training programs for health professionals and paraprofessionals.

France

The French health system is a prototype of Western European continental health systems. Its distinguishing feature of health care organization is the coexistence of a public and a private sector, both of which are largely financed collectively.[2] Its underlying structure rests on an uneasy truce between the medical profession and the French state, which remains guided by three principles: solidarity, pluralism, and liberal medicine.

The principle of *solidarity* is rooted in a belief in mutual aid and cooperation. It suggests that health insurance is a right for all—sick and well, high and low income, active and inactive—and that social security payroll contributions ought to be calculated on the basis of ability to pay, not of anticipated risk.[3] The principle of *pluralism* suggests that there should be room for a diversity of health insurance schemes and modes of health care delivery. It also suggests that the state ought not to meddle with the traditional prerogatives of various interest groups. Finally, the principle of *liberal medicine* suggests that physicians should be free to practice on a fee-for-service basis, that patients should be free to choose their physicians, that physicians should be assured clinical freedom, and that professional confidentiality should be respected.

Since these principles, like those guiding the American health system, are not necessarily consistent with one another, the structure of the French health sector, too, reflects the impact of often contradictory health policies.[4] In the name of solidarity, the French state has actively intervened in the health sector. Virtually the entire population (98 percent) is covered under national health insurance; there is an impressive public health program, particularly in the area of maternal and infant care; and there is a large and prestigious public hospital sector. Yet there is no country in the world, with the possible exception of the United States, in which the organization and commitment to private practice is more established than in France. Like the American Medical Association, French medical associations are monopolistic and scornful of state intrusion into their affairs. In France, as in the United States, there is a large and powerful proprietary hospital sector.

QUÉBEC

The Québec health system reflects a curious mix of American-style federalism and pragmatism and French-style centralism and government regulation. Its current structure reflects three central ideas: acceptance of the Canadian universal and comprehensive NHI program at the federal level; recognition that broad health goals ought to guide health policy; and commitment to developing primary care and promoting regionalization of health services.

Until recently the organization of medical care in Québec, like that in other Canadian provinces today, resembled that of the United States. Marmor and his collaborators have observed that

> Politically, socially, economically and culturally, the United States is closer to Canada than to any other nation. Canadian political authority is decentralized. Its tradition of dispute over federal power resembles the United States. The structure of the health industry is strikingly similar. . . . American hospitals and Canadian hospitals are largely "voluntary" and physicians in both countries are still typically paid under a fee-for-service system. The two countries similarly adjusted to the growth of health insurance, which was largely private, at first, becoming increasingly public in the postwar period.[5]

Beginning in 1970, however, health care reform in Québec, unlike that in other Canadian provinces and in the United States, took a dramatic turn. As Marc Renaud put it, "To what has been described as the science of muddling through, Québec seems to have opposed the strategy of global, almost irreversible, purposive legislative planning."[6] It was carried out in the French style of global reorganization by government decree and ministerial circular. The result has been to increase the power of the provincial government and to entirely reorganize the health sector. Since the creation of England's National Health Service in 1948, no social democracy has taken health care reform as far as has Québec.

ENGLAND

In contrast to the health systems in France and Québec, which may be described as modified market models of health resource allocation, the English National Health Service (NHS) is the model par excellence of a nationalized health system. In the modified market model, the allocation of health resources is largely determined by individual decisions acting through a regulated market. In the nationalized model, the allocation of resources is largely determined at a central level by the state. Michael Cooper indicates that after nationalization in England,

> health care was no longer rationed amongst competing claims by the willingness and ability to pay a market clearing price. Instead, the state accepted responsibility for ensuring that sufficient resources were made available to meet society's needs as defined and assessed by the medical and allied professions.[7]

The creation of the NHS in 1948 represents the most sweeping health care reform of any Western liberal democracy. Yet it may also be interpreted as an evolutionary step in a process of health sector transformation that had begun as early as 1911, when Lloyd George led the passage of the National Health Insurance Act.

After 1911, numerous commissions called for greater coordination through restructuring of the English health system. In 1920 the Dawson Report stressed the importance of regionalization.[8] In 1926 the Royal Commission on National Health Insurance advised extending health insurance coverage and reorganizing the health system with financing from general revenue funds.[9] In 1938 the British Medical Association (BMA) issued a report that also recommended the extension of health insurance coverage and urged better coordination of hospitals.[10] Finally, in 1942 the recommendations of the Beveridge Report stated that

> a comprehensive national health service will ensure for every citizen that there is available whatever medical treatment he

requires, in whatever form he requires it, domiciliary or institutional, general, specialist or consultant, and will ensure also the provision of dental, ophthalmic, and surgical appliances, nursery and midwifery and rehabilitation after accidents.[11]

During World War II, the coalition government's direction over the Emergency Medical Service led the government to prepare a plan for comprehensive health services that was even more far-reaching than the Beveridge Report. In addition, the BMA Medical Planning Commission prepared a blueprint for postwar change that advocated continuation of government central planning, expansion of regional arrangements devised by the coalition government, and development of health centers in which general practitioners (GPs) would practice.[12]

Odin Anderson has described the creation of the NHS as a rather broad change, logical in the British context because of the historic influence of "aristocratic *noblesse oblige* and Christian Socialism."[13] Vicente Navarro suggests that although the creation of the NHS represented a "victory for the working class," it was hardly revolutionary because it consolidated traditional class divisions between GPs and specialists within the medical sector.[14] Whether one agrees with Anderson or Navarro or with both (they are not necessarily contradictory), it is clear that nationalization entirely changed the institutional structure of the English health system.

The new NHS reflected three goals: equity, rationality, and professional autonomy. Conceived by Aneurin Bevan, chief architect of the NHS and minister of health, as the challenge of "generalizing the best," equity resulted in the elimination of financial barriers to medical care. Rationality provided the justification for a centralized administrative structure responsive to planning and government control. And the goal of professional autonomy led to a health system characterized by the free choice of doctors by patients and vice versa, elements of private practice, and a tripartite structure that preserved the traditional separation between GPs, public health workers, and hospital-based consultants.

FINANCING AND ORGANIZATION

THE UNITED STATES

Although there is no NHI program in the United States, roughly 30 percent of health expenditures are financed by private insurers. Four out of five Americans under the age of 65 have private health insurance coverage for inpatient services of both hospitals and physicians. This market for private health insurance is shared between commercial carriers, Blue Cross and Blue Shield plans. Blue Cross plans reimburse hospitals; Blue Shield plans reimburse physicians. As for government, federal and state contributions represent 40 percent of health care expenditures. The federal share of these expenditures is administered largely by the Health Care Financing Administration (HCFA).

Medicare and Medicaid are financed and administered quite differently. Medicare is a federal program for the elderly and the severely disabled. It is financed on the basis of Social Security taxes, as well as general revenue taxes and premiums paid by the beneficiaries. Medicaid, by contrast, is administered by the states. It is a program for the very poor financed primarily by federal and state general revenues. Blue Cross and Blue Shield plans as well as commercial insurers, are most often financed by employer and employee premiums. Although individuals are able to purchase insurance at high rates, most private insurance is purchased on a group basis. In the past, employers generally bargained with a third party payer to provide their employees a single insurance policy. At the present time there is a trend for employers to give their employees a choice between several competing health insurance plans.

Roughly two-thirds of all hospital beds in the United States are in private, including nonprofit or voluntary hospitals and proprietary hospitals that constitute 15 percent of the private beds. The other third of all hospital beds in the United States fall within the public sector—at the federal, state, county, and municipal levels of government. The federal government owns and operates separate hospital services for all military personnel and dependents; it also operates the Veterans Administration hospital system. State governments normally own and operate long-term care psychiatric hospitals; and individual counties and/or municipalities usually own and operate local public hospitals for those without insurance coverage, as well as those who are covered by Medicare and Medicaid.

Ambulatory care in the United States is provided largely by general practitioners and specialists in private office-based practice, either as solo practitioners, in small or large multispecialty groups or, to a lesser extent, in hospital out-patient departments and in hospital emergency rooms. It is primarily the poor and minorities in urban areas who use hospitals as their primary source of ambulatory care. In addition, there are local neighborhood health centers (NHCs) in most urban areas and a network of dispensaries for public health services including, in some cases, primary care. The NHCs were first organized in response to federal programs in the sixties. Now many of them are self-supporting or financed by nonprofit organizations and local and/or state governments. The dispensaries for public health services fall under the responsibility of local governments but often receive federal subsidies to organize such prevention programs as maternal and child health, hypertension screening, and immunizations.

Unlike the tradition in European countries such as France and England, office-based private practitioners in the United States are accorded hospital admitting privileges since they are responsible for most admissions to the voluntary and proprietary hospitals. Only the public hospitals and the university owned or controlled teaching hospitals have full time salaried physicians on most of the hospital services.

A notable innovation in the organization of ambulatory care in the United States is the prepaid group practice—a group of physicians usually working together with a group of hospitals, all of which agree to enroll a population in the new organization and to accept a prepaid fee for each member instead of the conventional mode of billing on a fee-for-service basis. The most widely known form of prepaid group practice is the Kaiser-Permanente Health Plan, labeled in the 1970s as a health maintenance organization (HMO). Physicians working in HMOs may be reimbursed on a fee-for-service basis or they may work on a salary basis with the possibility of earning a yearly bonus depending on the organization's success at providing the full range of necessary medical services, but with far lower rates of hospital admission than in fee-for-service practice. At present, there are roughly 240 HMOs in the United States, which have a total membership of 9 million, roughly 4 percent of the population.

FRANCE

French employers and employees contribute compulsory payroll taxes to the social security system and, in return, all employees and dependents are entitled to comprehensive medical care coverage. Of the total population, 76 percent is covered under the National Health Insurance Fund for Salaried Workers,[15] the CNAMTS.* Agricultural workers (9 percent) and the self-employed (7 percent) have their own health insurance program, and another 6 percent of the population is covered under special welfare programs administered by the Ministry of Health.

Roughly two-thirds of all hospital beds in France, including all university and regional specialty hospitals, are public and fall under the administration of the Ministry of Health. Of the total number of hospital beds in the private (volun-

*Caisse Nationale d'Assurance Maladie des Travailleurs Salariés.

tary) sector, over one-half are in proprietary hospitals known as *cliniques*; the remainder are in private nonprofit hospitals.

The private nonprofit hospitals are similar to the public hospitals in their bed capacity and service mix. The cliniques are quite different, however. The average clinique has thirty-eight beds, whereas the average public hospital has 240 beds.[16] Cliniques have only 10 percent of all medical beds and almost half of all surgical and obstetric beds. In short, in comparison to hospitals, cliniques tend to be smaller and to handle easier cases, especially maternity and routine surgery, leaving the public sector with serious cases requiring prolonged hospitalization and capital-intensive therapy. In terms of organizational strategy, cliniques have served as an institution within which the medical profession has retained control over its own work outside the bureaucratic structures of the public sector.

Ambulatory care in France is provided largely by general practitioners or specialists in private (solo or group) practice, in public hospital outpatient departments, or in hospital emergency rooms. In addition, there are dispensaries that provide public health services and a small network of health centers, sometimes attached to the dispensaries, which provide primary care. These establishments are usually set up and managed by municipalities, mutual aid funds, or local health insurance funds.

Seventy percent of French physicians work in private practice, whereas 30 percent are fully salaried; but roughly half of the 70 percent also work on part-time salaries, mostly in public hospitals, dispensaries, and health centers, and in the area of occupational health.

General practitioners and specialists in France are free to set up practice wherever they like. And consumers are free to choose their physicians. Upon visiting their physicians, consumers pay the full charge of their visit. In return, the physician gives them a receipt to present to their local health insurance fund, either by mail or in person. The fund then reimburses the consumer 75 percent of the charges as set in

a national fee schedule. The remaining 25 percent represents a consumer co-payment which the French call a *ticket
modérateur*.

In general, the size of the co-payment depends on the
kind of medical service consumed. For most laboratory
tests, dental care, and drug prescriptions, the co-payment is
30 percent; for specially designated or particularly expensive drugs it is 20 percent; and for hospital services it is 20
percent unless the hospital stay exceeds thirty days or
requires costly therapy for prolonged illnesses such as dia-
betes, polio, and cancer, in which case medical care is free of
charge to the consumer.

QUÉBEC

In contrast to the French system, in Québec the entire
population is covered under one NHI program. Roughly
half the cost is financed by the federal government out of
general revenues, and the other half is financed by the
provincial government and allocated to the Québec Health
Insurance Board (QHIB).*

The QHIB is a public corporation that includes representatives from business, labor, health professions, hospitals, consumer groups, and the provincial government. Its
mandate is to administer the NHI program and to make
payments to health professionals and hospitals for all services rendered. But the Ministry of Social Affairs is responsible for major policy decisions affecting the QHIB, including negotiations with the health professions.

In contrast to the French system, coverage for drugs and
dental services is more limited. Most health care, however, is
free at the point of consumption. The consumer has merely
to present a plastic charge card known as *la castonquette*

*Régie de l'Assurance Maladie du Québec.

(named after Claude Castonguay, minister of social affairs in 1970), and the providers are reimbursed by the QHIB.

Over 90 percent of hospital beds in Québec are, strictly speaking, in the voluntary, private, nonprofit sector. Because they are almost entirely financed by the government, hospitals in Québec are usually considered to be public institutions. They differ from French public hospitals in two respects. First, the physicians who work in Québec's hospitals, like their colleagues in the United States, are generally not salaried. Second, the hospitals are managed by private associations known as corporations that are subject to more flexible administrative controls and not bound by civil service regulations.

Ambulatory care in Québec is provided by physicians in office-based private solo practice, in private polyclinics, or in any one of eighty-one Local Health and Social Service Centers (CLSCs).* The CLSCs, which correspond closely to what Henrik Blum calls the Primary Well-Being Center,[17] represent Québec's exceptional experiment in community health. As local organizations charged with developing their own health and social programs, they provide counseling services, primary health and social services, and referral services to secondary and tertiary levels of care when required. At present, they provide only a small fraction of the ambulatory care provided in Québec, the bulk of these services still being provided by office-based physicians.

In addition to the CLSCs, there are thirty-two Departments of Community Health (DSCs)† that provide basic public health services. Although they are located within hospitals, most of their activities do not involve patients. They conduct epidemiological studies and devise health prevention and promotion strategies for their target populations.

*Centres Locaux de Services Communautaires.
†Département de Santé Communautaire.

ENGLAND

When the NHS was established, virtually all voluntary
hospitals were nationalized and, together with municipal
hospitals, placed under the control of the Ministry of
Health. The ministry delegated responsibility for hospitals
to three authorities: regional hospital boards (RHBs), hospital management committees, (HMCs), and boards of
governors (BGs). The RHBs were responsible for supervising hospitals within each of fourteen hospital regions.
Hospitals were grouped under roughly twenty to thirty
HMCs that were responsible to the minister of health via the
RHB for hospital management and preparation of annual
budget estimates. Finally, because of a concession by
Aneurin Bevan to the Royal Colleges of Physicians and
Surgeons, thirty-six BGs were established to administer the
more prestigious teaching hospitals. The BGs were directly
responsible to the Ministry of Health.

A compromise with consultants (hospital physicians) in
1948 resulted in the continuation of two forms of private
hospital practice in England: so-called pay beds within NHS
hospitals and private hospitals outside the NHS. Pay beds
amount to just over 1 percent of all NHS beds and 2 percent
of all nonpsychiatric cases handled in the NHS. The number of private hospital beds outside the NHS is growing but
still negligible compared with the number of pay beds
within NHS hospitals. For both pay beds and private hospital beds, roughly one out of twenty-five people is covered by
private insurance; but total expenditures for private medical care by insurance come to just over 1 percent of national
expenditures of the NHS.[18] As in France, patients tend to
use private facilities for routine procedures rather than for
complex therapy and long-term care. But in England a
large proportion of private practice caters to the unmet
demand within NHS hospitals. Since the NHS operates on a
zero-price system, rationing of need by medical criteria has
resulted in waiting lists for appointments with specialists as
well as for certain categories of inpatient admissions.[19]

Thus, the private sector provides a mechanism for queue jumping.

Ambulatory care in the NHS is organized around the office-based GP, who serves as gatekeeper to the hospital system. After the creation of the NHS, health care was provided free of charge at the point of consumption and *all* residents in England were eligible to register on any GP's patient list. Executive councils were formed to administer general medical, dental, pharmaceutical, and ophthalmic services; local health authorities were nationalized and continued to provide a range of public health services including home nursing and home help.

More than 95 percent of the population is now registered with GPs and roughly 90 percent of GPs practice predominantly within the NHS. Three-fifths work in groups of three to seven, and nearly a quarter work in health centers provided by the NHS. The maximum GP list size is 3,500, and the average is just over 2,300 and falling. GPs have an unchallenged right not to accept every patient and, in theory, patients are free to change GPs; but collectively, GPs have agreed that all patients will be accepted by someone.

PROVIDER REIMBURSEMENT

The United States

Hospitals in the United States are reimbursed through a variety of mechanisms ranging from fee-for-service charges, to per-case rates, to a capitation system whereby the institution receives a fixed amount for each enrolled member. The most common reimbursement mechanism is when the hospital is paid on the basis of per diem costs. Generally, the method of hospital reimbursement is the outcome of formal agreements between hospitals and third-party payers.

Most hospitals use charges as one method of obtaining payment. This applies for commercial insurance companies, most Blue Cross plans, and patients responsible for all or part of their bill (e.g., that part not covered by a third party). By far, the most important source of revenue to hospitals is based upon retrospectively determined per diem costs. This is the method adopted by Medicare and until 1982, by almost all state Medicaid programs. There are, of course, differences in the amounts paid to hospitals based on differences in cost (e.g., urban areas have higher costs than rural areas) but the same factors are taken into account in what is considered an allowable cost.

The determination of per diem costs has been a source of frequent debate between accountants working for hospitals and those employed by third-party payers. The main issue centers around what constitutes reasonable costs: teaching, research, depreciation, bad debts? But there is general agreement that cost-based reimbursement provides financial incentives for hospitals and their physicians to expand the volume and intensity of service provision. Hospital administrators have found that they must "game" the reimbursement system to obtain maximum revenues. Moreover, since health insurance coverage for hospital care is more extensive and universal than insurance for primary care, there is an added incentive to perform certain procedures on an inpatient hospital basis rather than in private practice.

As for ambulatory care outside the hospital, the predominant form of payment for physician services is fee-for-service whereby the physician receives a fee for each separately identifiable service rendered.[20] There are two major methods of determining how much to pay physicians for specific procedures: fee schedules and the usual, customary, and reasonable charge (UCR) system. Fee schedules specify a list of allowable fees for specific medical procedures. They are used by twenty-six state Medicaid programs, about half of the Blue Shield plans, and many commercial insurers. The UCR system is used by Medicare, twenty-four state Medicaid programs, half of the Blue Shield plans, and some commercial insurers. Under the

UCR system, reimbursement for particular medical procedures is calculated statistically from actual physician billings, based on the "reasonable charge" that is the lowest of (1) the physician's billed charge, (2) the physician's customary charge for that procedure, and (3) the prevailing charge (in the geographic area) for the procedure.

Like the method of hospital reimbursement, this system of physician reimbursement has had powerful cost-generating effects. To begin with, it has allowed physician expenditures to grow at an annual rate exceeding 15 percent. It has also favored the development of technology-intensive diagnostic, laboratory, radiological, and surgical procedures. Moreover, it has encouraged inpatient hospital procedures instead of ambulatory-based and primary-care services. For example, on an hourly basis, surgical procedures are generally compensated at rates two to three times those of primary-care visits.

FRANCE

As in the United States, public hospitals in France are reimbursed by the CNAMTS on the basis of costs incurred. The patient day is the principal unit of reimbursement. Its price is calculated by dividing total operating expenditures, including teaching and research costs and a range of ancillary services, by the total number of patient days. Since all public hospital physicians are on salaries, as individuals they have no financial incentives to increase the number of medical procedures. From the point of view of the hospital manager, however, there is an incentive to extend the length of stays in order to increase hospital revenues. In the cliniques, the patient day is less of a catchall category because most services and medical procedures are billed separately on a fee-for-service basis according to annually negotiated rates. But, unlike the public hospitals, physicians are reimbursed directly on a fee-for-service basis for all medical procedures performed on their patients. Thus, there is a built-in incentive to maximize "throughput" and also to generously perform medical procedures. To sum up, reimbursement incentives in France tend to encourage hospital-based care.

As far as ambulatory care is concerned, the CNAMTS reimburses physicians in private practice on the basis of a fee schedule that is negotiated annually between physician associations and the CNAMTS. Like all fee-for-service reimbursement systems, there is an incentive at the margin for physicians to multiply the number of medical procedures performed in order to increase their income. But the more serious problem is that the relative weights of the fee schedule are not annually readjusted to account for changes in technology that result in economies of scale in such areas as the production of laboratory tests and radiological examinations. Consequently, such price distortions have tended to encourage high-technology medical procedures.

The CNAMTS not only negotiates reimbursement rates with health professionals and private hospitals; it also finances 70 percent of aggregate health expenditures and contributes roughly 30 percent of the capital for hospital construction. Thus, its implicit policies are critical in determining the structure of resource allocation in the health sector.

QUÉBEC

Hospitals in Québec, unlike those of France and the United States, are no longer paid on the basis of per diem hospital costs; they are financed on the basis of closed budgets (*budgets globaux*) allocated by the Ministry of Social Affairs after approval from the treasury. The hospital budget covers all operating costs excluding capital expenditures, construction costs, financial charges, research subsidies, and physician remuneration. Physicians are reimbursed directly on a fee-for-service basis by the QHIB.

Although hospital administrators have an inducement to minimize costs, physicians have a financial incentive to perform medical procedures not merely for hospitalized patients but also for outpatient clients. After a physician's gross income reaches $100,000, however, he is reimbursed at only 25 percent of the fee schedule rate. This policy is intended both to control physician income and to reduce the growing number of medical procedures that are often of marginal benefit to patients.

For ambulatory services, the QHIB directly reimburses all health professionals. In the CLSCs, the QHIB remunerates physicians on a salaried basis. The starting salary is roughly $35,000 for a thirty-five-hour week. In private practice the QHIB reimburses physicians (in solo practice and polyclinics) on a fee-for-service basis. As in France, the fee schedule is negotiated annually among physician associations, the QHIB, and the Ministry of Social Affairs. Like the French fee schedule, Québec's fee schedule also has built-in incentives favoring the use of technology based medical procedures. In contrast to France, however, general practitioners are paid the same as specialists for identical procedures and are reimbursed based on the length of time taken by the procedure. Verification of billings is more assiduously pursued than in France, and more rigorous quality control procedures have been introduced. This is partly because information on patient diagnoses is collected by the QHIB, whereas in France it is regarded as confidential.

ENGLAND

As in Québec, hospitals in England are financed on the basis of closed budgets. As in France, consultants are remunerated on a salaried basis. While roughly 70 percent of consultants work part-time, about half of these are remunerated on the basis of "maximum part-time": four and one-half days a week. Although private practice is a popular and lucrative activity, it is nevertheless marginal in

terms of aggregate physician income. According to a 1971 –
1972 survey, the average income of part-timers was 18
percent higher than that of full-timers.[21]

As for the GPs, since the passage of national health insurance in 1911, they have been remunerated largely on the
basis of capitation payments. After the creation of the NHS,
the executive councils kept lists of patients enrolled with
GPs and paid fees to these independent contractors based
on the number of enrolled patients. Capitation payments,
like salaries, are negotiated centrally between professional
associations and the Ministry of Health. In addition to these
payments, which vary according to patient age, GPs have
received an increasing portion of their income in the form
of noncapitation payments. For example, they receive
"basic practice allowances" depending on where they set up
practice. Further, roughly 3 percent of GP income is
derived from fee-for-service payment for such designated
services as home visits and night calls.

Both hospital and ambulatory care in England compared
with France and Québec, represent a far more controlled
system of provider reimbursement based largely on fixed
payments that are independent of the cost and volume of
services rendered. One of the effects of such a system is the
"dumping problem." Although GPs have no incentive to
multiply the number of medical procedures performed,
they are perhaps too often inclined to refer their patients to
outpatient hospital consultants. Such referrals have no
doubt contributed both to the size of waiting lists and to the
length of waiting times. In addition, they have contributed
to promoting "hospital-centered health care."[22] Between
1951 and 1975, hospital care increased from 55.7 to 65.8
percent of health expenditures, whereas general medical
services decreased from 9.5 to 6.1 percent of total health
expenditures.[23]

Contrary to frequent fears among physicians in the
United States, elimination of fee-for-service reimbursement in England did not decrease the power of the medical
profession. Consultants and GPs have complete clinical

freedom, lifelong contracts, and a powerful role in the formation of public policy.[24] Moreover, they are not subject to the kinds of medical audits and quality control procedures that are emerging in France, Québec, and the United States.[25] Salary negotiations with the government have often been tough and embittered, and some groups (e.g., GPs in the fifties and consultants in the seventies) have suffered income cuts.[26] Although by international standards, physician income in England is relatively low (table 7), by English wage standards, the situation has not significantly deteriorated since Aneurin Bevan claimed that he "choked [the consultants'] mouths with gold" in order to get the National Health Service Act passed.[27]

TABLE 7

DOCTORS' INCOME IN RELATION TO GDP PER HEAD AND EARNED INCOME, 1974 OR NEAR DATE

	Percentages	
	Ratio of doctors' income to:	
	Per capita income (GDP per head)	Average production worker's gross earnings
Canada	6.8	4.8
Denmark (1973)	5.7	3.8
Finland (1970)	5.2	4.2
France	7.0	7.0
Germany (1973)	8.5	6.1
Ireland (1973)	7.6	3.5
Italy (1973)	9.5	6.8
Netherlands (1973)	10.2	6.3
Norway	3.4	2.4
Sweden	4.6	3.5
United Kingdom (1973)	4.5	2.7
United States	6.7	5.6

Source: Adapted from table 9 in *Public Expenditure on Health* (Paris: OECD Studies in Resource Allocation, July, 1977).

5

Health Planning under National Health
Insurance: France

The French economy combines elements of a centralized
étatist tradition with those of private entrepreneurship and
big business. In textbooks on economics France is known
for its "indicative" planning.[1] On the one hand, this is a
political process by which choices are made about the allocation of future resources; on the other, it is a technical
process that relies on market research and macroeconomic
models to improve information for decision-making.
Health planning in France takes place within this system of
national economic planning that has attracted the attention
of planners around the world.

Following World War II, a national planning commission
(CGP)* was created as part of a broad set of measures to
strengthen the role of the state in the control and direction
of economic development. The CGP, however, had no
power of direct command. As Commissioner Pierre Massé
described it,

> The role of the planning commission inside the administrative
> and governmental machinery is confined to that of proposing,
> advising and estimating. It takes part in discussions and pre-
> pares decisions, but it manages no funds and has itself no
> power of economic intervention. No department or ministry

*Commissariat Général du Plan.

can reasonably fear to see it encroach on its field; but it provides the administration as a whole with the opportunity of coordinating its schemes and solving its conflicts on neutral ground.[2]

To implement the plan, French policymakers make use of centralized administrative controls over the public sector and selected incentives and regulations for the private sector.

Since 1946 the CGP has produced eight plans for social and economic development. Work is currently in progress on the ninth. The plans, intended to be explicit, consistent, and comprehensive, are the outcome of a broadly based representative process. But there have been problems in implementing the social goals of the plans. This is owing largely to two factors. First, actual economic policy tends to react to short-term pressures rather than to long-term planning considerations. Second, as Stephen Cohen has shown, the choice of which portions of the plan to implement is usually a result of decisions taken by an elite group forming an alliance between big business and the state.[3] This alliance succeeded in modernizing French industry and creating a new industrial base in aerospace, automobiles, nuclear energy, and computers. The social goals of the plans, however, have consistently called for redistributive policies and social investments over which planners had virtually no control.[4]

Health planning in France reflects all the problems of national economic planning. The formal process of preparing health plans is organized by the CGP. It is a broadly based process in which representative interests and selected specialists participate. But the actual policies that are implemented have usually been developed by the Ministry of Health and the National Health Insurance Fund for Salaried Workers (CNAMTS)* on the basis of negotiation with health industry representatives (e.g., hospital and physician associations).

*Caisse Nationale d'Assurance Maladie des Travailleurs Salariés.

Rather than exploring the evolution of health planning in the context of formal national economic plans, it is more fruitful to view French health planning as pragmatic state intervention in the health sector. The actual role of health planning has been to help steer the process of change, first during the relative boom of the fifties and sixties and then during the recession of the seventies and beginning of the eighties. During both of these periods, French health planners wavered between protecting the interests of private medical practice on a fee-for-service basis—what the French call *la médecine libérale*—and adapting the health sector to technological and economic imperatives. During the first phase, health planners largely succeeded in constructing new hospitals and modernizing old ones. During the second phase, in spite of notable efforts to rationalize the allocation of resources, they have failed, as yet, to implement health plans and, above all, to contain the growth of health care costs.

ORIGINS OF HEALTH PLANNING

The first national health insurance (NHI) bill in France was passed in 1928 and it covered 14 percent of the population.[5] Following passage of this bill, physicians promptly recognized the leading question on the health policy agenda: what would be the role of third-party payers in attaching conditions about the way in which their money was spent by physicians?

As early as 1929, in a letter to the minister of labor, Paul Cibrie, who was the first secretary general of the first physicians' trade union, Confédération des Syndicats Médicaux Français (CSMF), expressed concern over the emergence of third-party payment:

> The medical profession is under no illusions about the consequences of the contractual liberty allowed for under the Law. We understand administrative procedure well enough to know that the [health insurance] funds will want to impose

allowable charges and third-party payment. And we have
great difficulty identifying an impartial institution capable of
arbitrating between the opposing positions of the medical profession and that of the health insurance funds.[6]

Cibrie's concern was well warranted. He anticipated what
French policymakers did not realize until 1960—that NHI
and the right of physicians to set their own fees are incom-
patible. Any NHI program leads quickly to a system of
national reimbursement controls. The aims, initially, are to
control costs and to eliminate abuse; but soon there are
other functions—for example, to conduct epidemiological
studies and to plan for health care needs including the
extension of health insurance.

The next step in this direction was the Social Security
Ordinance. It was enacted immediately following World
War II (1945) in the spirit of national solidarity expressed at
Liberation. This ordinance provided for pensions and
family benefits and also called for universal NHI. The
process of extending health insurance coverage to the
entire French population has taken over thirty years to
complete. In 1960 only 75 percent of the population was
insured. But in 1961 benefits were extended to agricultural
workers raising coverage to 88 percent; in 1965 most of the
remaining self-employed population such as shopkeepers,
artisans, students, and professionals in private practice were
progressively brought into the system. And in 1978 a law
was passed that entitled the entire population to join the
NHI program.

Until 1960, French physicians in private practice re-
mained free to set their own fees. With the ministerial
decree of May 12, however, President Charles de Gaulle
created a system of annual individual contracts with price
ceilings and uniform fees. By giving individual physicians
the choice of whether to remain eligible for reimbursement
by NHI funds and consequently abide by nationally set fees,
the government struck a severe blow to the CSMF. This
strategic move produced irreconcilable conflict within the
medical profession. Strong partisans of la médecine libérale

in Paris, Lyon, and along the Riviera, refused to abide by the negotiated fees and formed a rival trade union, the Fédération des Médecins de France (FMF). Nonetheless, by 1964, 80 percent of French physicians, including most members of the FMF, were participating in the NHI program.[7]

Another policy issue involved control and governance of the health insurance funds. The original founders of the French NHI program established in 1945 believed that regional and local funds should be managed by elected representatives. But this did not provide the government with the degree of central control that it wanted over the funds. Thus, in 1967, a major reform of the entire social security system was enacted. The government created three predominant national funds within the social security system: health insurance including maternity, invalidity, and industrial accidents; family benefits; and pensions. Each fund was given a certain autonomy to manage its finances and responsibility for balancing its budget. In addition, the local and regional funds were placed under the administrative authority of the national system. Governance of the national funds was divided between representatives of workers (trade unions) and of employers (the Confédération Nationale du Patronat Français—CNPF). With French trade unions divided and the CNPF united, power has actually rested in a partnership between the CNPF and the state. The current Socialist government of François Mitterand proposes to change this and restore some form of electoral process but as of January 1983 there has been no reform.

In 1967 the CNAMTS became the principal payer for health care services. This action resulted in the kind of countervailing power that the physicians' trade unions feared most. For once their reimbursement came principally from one source, there was always the threat that such competing modes of medical practice as health centers would be financed by that source. In fact, the CNAMTS has agreed not to compete with la médecine libérale by establishing its own health centers for the provision of primary care. It has also extended health insurance benefits to all physicians. In return, in 1971 the physicians' trade unions signed a national collective contract with the government and the CNAMTS. They agreed to accept reimbursement rates negotiated annually on the basis of a national fee schedule.[8] The rates apply to all physicians in private practice with the exception of those who individually take the initiative to opt out.

Since 1928 when the first French health insurance bill was passed, there have been periodic conflicts within the medical profession and between physicians' trade unions and the state over the conditions of medical practice under health insurance.[9] Henri Hatzfeld argues that these conflicts have resulted in the taming of the French medical profession.[10] Others, including physicians, even speak of proletarianization insofar as conditions of medical practice have been substantially altered.[11] Still another point of view, albeit a minority one, is that the medical fraternity continues to dominate health policy but that physician associations, themselves, will soon demand a shift from fee-for-service to salary reimbursement.[12] These issues are explosive. But there is a growing consensus that

> the physician appears condemned to lose a part of his professional autonomy: his income will no longer be determined by his freedom to set charges and by his success; he will become a man employed on a salary based on status or a man hired on contract; his place in social organization will become more precise, more established.[13]

Dr. Cibrie's concern about the threatening potential of third-party payment proved accurate. Since 1971, the CNAMTS has begun considering ways in which to monitor the utilization of health services and the prescribing patterns of physicians. Such activities portend the ways in which billing information, and potentially reimbursement incentives, can be used to reform the organization of health services under a system of NHI. The more decisive health planning initiatives, however, have come directly from the government itself.

HEALTH PLANNING AS HOSPITAL CONSTRUCTION
AND MODERNIZATION

In contrast to the gradual transformation of la médecine libérale, French hospitals were abruptly reorganized. Following World War II, just as big business formed a partnership with the state to modernize industry, so too an elite group of physicians and the leaders of the public hospital association—the barons of the health sector—collaborated with the Ministry of Health to plan for rapid reform of French hospitals.

In 1956 a selectively chosen task force was appointed under the direction of the distinguished pediatrician Robert Debré. Its recommendations led to the first significant piece of health planning legislation: the Hospital Reform Act, passed in 1958 under de Gaulle, when Dr. Debré's son was prime minister.[14] This legislation merged university medical schools with the best-equipped public hospital facilities. The new institution, called a CHU (Centre Hospitalier Universitaire), was assigned the responsibility for providing high technology medicine and superspecialty services to regions with populations of over one million. As with Regional Medical Programs in the United States, an important effect of the Hospital Reform Act was to consolidate and control the diffusion of high technology medicine and reduce the gap between biomedical knowledge and its application.

Another effect of the Hospital Reform Act was to initiate a shift from fee-for-service toward salary reimbursement of hospital-based physicians. During the legislative debates on the proposed reform, the medical profession opposed the bill on the grounds that the shift in reimbursement mechanism would gradually turn all physicians into civil servants. Some of the younger physicians, however, supported the reform. As early as 1957, Dr. Jacques Monier, the president of the CSMF, had urged his colleagues to support the proposed bill. "Comprenez-vous," he once asked of them, "qu'il est impossible que vous restiez complètement individualistes dans une société qui est en train de s'organiser sur le plan collectif?"[15] Nevertheless, the highest ranking clinical professors, les grands patrons, resisted vigorously and succeeded in conserving that part of la médecine libérale they considered most dear: the right to hospitalize their private, paying patients in "private beds" within their service at the public hospital.[16]

Beginning with the second national economic plan (1954–1957), reconstruction was far enough along in the industrial sector so that the CGP could begin assessing needs for construction of new hospitals and modernization of old ones. The major health planning efforts, however, were centered within the Ministry of Health. The ministry is a centralized bureaucracy that carries out parliamentary intent as interpreted by an elite group of technically competent civil servants: technocrats. Planning tasks and methods are determined in Paris. Local and regional public health administrations, the DDASS and the DRASS,* execute ministerial circulars. For example, the ministry specifies procedures for making resource inventories and passes down criteria for purposes of estimating need. The DDASS and DRASS send up the necessary information along with their own budget requests. Thus, social priorities, as perceived by the health technocrats and their coalition of health care providers, are implemented while broad participation organized by the CGP is kept from hobbling the planning process.

Since 1959, flurries of ministerial circulars have periodically reclassified the public hospital system into finer categories based on criteria such as spatial service areas, functions performed, types of personnel employed, availability of specialized medical services, and average lengths of patient stays. Such classification schemes have forced recognition of the multiple goals and functions of a hierarchy of health institutions by distinguishing such roles as

---

*Direction Départementale des Affaires Sanitaires et Sociales; Direction Régionale des Affaires Sanitaires et Sociales.

diagnosis, therapy, prevention, teaching, and research. Each time these categories were delineated anew, the Ministry of Health called for updated hospital bed resource inventories, and the planning of more hospital construction followed.

Throughout the 1960s, while the Ministry of Health was distributing capital funds for public hospital construction and modernization, the CNAMTS was making an indirect but critical contribution to the private proprietary hospital industry. Until 1968, the CNAMTS negotiated per diem hospital fees for cliniques on the basis of equivalent rates for the closest public hospital. Cliniques, however, have consistently handled easy cases—especially maternity care and routine surgery—leaving the public sector with the serious medical cases requiring prolonged hospitalization and capital-intensive care. By law, a public hospital must also be open twenty-four hours a day, must keep its occupancy rate under 95 percent, and must be equipped to handle all emergencies. Moreover, public hospitals include regional teaching hospitals engaging in biomedical research and medical training. For these reasons, average costs of public hospitals tend to be higher than equivalent costs of cliniques. Consequently, this system of provider reimbursement enabled the medical entrepreneur to skim the cream off the market. Thus, in the sixties, while public hospital costs rose faster than those in the private proprietary sector, cliniques were reaping profits from the CNAMTS, and their bed capacity grew at a faster rate than in the public sector.[17]

Since 1968, the government and the CNAMTS have tightened control over the terms of reimbursement for cliniques. Cliniques are no longer compared with the closest public hospital in determining their per diem rate. Health planners have devised more sophisticated techniques for classifying similar groups of cliniques and determining reasonable per diem fees. Also, the CNAMTS no longer allows increases in per diem rates for cliniques without prior authorization from the Ministry of Finance. As a result of these changes, in 1979, some banks no longer considered cliniques an attractive investment opportunity.[18] Nonetheless, the private sector has succeeded in expanding its bed capacity at a rate exceeding that of the public sector.[19] A major source of financing for cliniques came from removing as many procedures as possible from inclusion in the per diem rate of reimbursement by the CNAMTS. This practice explains the finding of Emile Lévy and others that the activity of cliniques is best characterized by the quest for both high revenues and long lengths of stay during which a large number of medical procedures are performed.[20]

By the mid-seventies, health planners in the Ministry of Health had succeeded in modernizing and expanding the capacity of French hospitals (table 8). But in the process of planning hospital construction and modernization, three new problems emerged. First, conflicts between public hospitals and cliniques surfaced. Second, disparities in the distribution of hospital beds, between as well as within geographic regions, provoked concern. Finally, the growth of health care expenditures threatened to get out of hand.

CONFLICTS BETWEEN PUBLIC HOSPITALS AND CLINIQUES

In 1963 cliniques represented 26.4 percent of all acute hospital beds; in 1978 they had grown to include 34.8 percent.[21] This growth in number of beds was accompanied by increasing ideological conflicts between public and private sectors and growing polarization between salaried medical specialists in public hospitals and physicians practicing in the cliniques on a fee-for-service basis.[22] Debates on the relative virtues of the private and public sectors have frequently been published in the press.[23] Associations of private cliniques have released studies showing the cliniques are managed more efficiently than hospitals and have argued that the state should consequently encourage the

TABLE 8
The Growth of Acute Care Hospital Beds in France 1963–1978

	1963			1968			1973			1975			1978		
	Public	Private	Total	Public	Private	Total	Public	Private	Total	Public	Private	Total	Public	Private	Total
Medical	119,000	12,085	131,085	129,239	16,334	145,573	143,696	24,913	168,609	143,328	28,283	171,611	129,639	31,814	161,453
Surgical	58,839	43,192	102,031	63,169	53,222	116,391	67,763	62,808	130,571	69,067	64,505	133,572	69,196	67,926	137,122
Maternity	15,861	14,325	30,185	16,331	15,355	31,686	16,133	15,262	31,395	16,360	14,549	30,909	18,964	13,965	32,929
Total	193,700	69,602	263,302	208,739	84,911	293,650	227,592	102,983	330,275	228,755	107,337	336,092	217,799	113,705	331,504

Source: J. de Kervasdoué, "La Politique de l'Etat en Matière d'Hospitalisation Privée. 1962–1978. Analyse des Conséquences de Mesures Contradictoires," *Annales Economiques de Clermont-Ferrand*, 16 (1980).

growth of the private sector.[24] Representatives of the public sector have reminded their private sector colleagues of the burdens of teaching, research, and high-cost illness, all of which must be borne by the public hospital. The state's chameleonlike response to these debates has led simultaneously to frequent denunciation of cliniques by public officials and to their rapid growth at public expense.

Though most medical technology and specialty care was, and still is, provided in the public hospitals, material conditions were far superior in the newly built cliniques. Prestigious public hospital buildings were dilapidated or obsolete in the fifties and sixties. Even in 1970, there were still 80,000 public hospital beds in bleak communal wards.[25] The public hospitals sought more beds and improvements in material conditions to "humanize" their environment. But despite the generally superior quality of medical care in the public sector, even the best public hospitals, such as those of l'Assistance Publique in Paris, were losing patients to the cliniques.[26]

DISPARITIES IN THE DISTRIBUTION OF HOSPITAL BEDS

In 1973, disparities in the distribution of public hospital beds between administrative regions ranged from 3.3 to 6.7 beds per 1,000 population.[27] The private sector only exacerbated this inequality, for it provided only 24 percent of hospital facilities in the poorest regions.[28]

Within regions, disparities in the distribution of hospital beds were also perceived to be a problem.[29] For example, for 62 percent of the population living in the four central sectors of the Paris region, there were 66 percent of the general hospital beds, 76 percent of the common specialty beds, and 87 percent of the highly specialized beds. For surgery, this concentration was even more extreme: 62 percent of the population was served by 66 percent of the general surgery beds, 83 percent of the common specialty beds, and 96 percent of the highly specialized beds.[30]

THE GROWTH OF HEALTH CARE EXPENDITURES

In 1965, during the preparation of the fifth national economic plan, the CGP became involved in health planning because rising national health expenditures could no longer be ignored in national economic planning. It is not surprising that the broadly based Commission on Social Transfers underscored national health insurance expenditures as a critical problem for the future and proposed rationalization policies for the health system in order to contain costs.[31]

Similar concerns influenced the Ministry of Health. Under the direction of Robert Boulin, a three-volume report was released outlining specific programs to rationalize resource allocation within the health sector.[32] Further, in 1969, a national task force released a report, *Reflections on the Future of the Health System*, which challenged the medical paradigm of hospital planning. In particular, it took exception to the dominant emphasis on therapeutic "engineering" techniques and biomedical research and the neglect of environmental and social aspects of illness. It advocated a regionalized health system that would develop primary care, link it to secondary- and tertiary-care centers, and encourage substitution of ambulatory care for inpatient hospital care.[33]

Along with Boulin's report, the task force underlined the need for concentrating more resources on "health promotion." It recommended a whole range of special programs—for example, to improve highway safety and emergency medical services and to reduce perinatal mortality, alcoholism, cancer, cardiovascular disease, and mental illness. It also proposed to reorganize the supply of health services by reforms that ranged from the promotion of group practice and greater use of paramedical personnel to improvements in hospital management techniques and direct coordination, as well as increased control over private and public sector growth.

By the end of the first decade of the Fifth Republic (1958 to 1968), the practice of health planning as hospital construction and modernization was no longer considered adequate by health planners. They proposed to regionalize and coordinate health service institutions and to allocate resources to enhance health and reduce the incidence of illness rather than devote disproportionate efforts to the growth and refinement of medical techniques. In short, health planners were proposing not merely to modernize; their aim now was rationalization to promote more effective and efficient resource allocation.

HEALTH PLANNING AS RATIONALIZATION

The response of the Ministry of Health to the drive for rationalization was to establish a new division charged with initiating PPBS-type studies—what the French call RCB*— to rationalize budget allocations.[34] Program budgets were devised and cost effectiveness studies were undertaken to assist policymakers in choosing intervention strategies. The studies included perinatality, highway safety, school health programs, infant care programs, flu vaccinations, and nurse training programs. The largest health program to emerge from this process was aimed at reducing perinatal mortality.[35]

Since 1970, the perinatal mortality rate has decreased considerably in France. Subsequent RCB studies, however, have been largely ignored, as those making budgetary decisions have responded more readily to political pressures than to the technical advice of health planners.[36] The division charged with planning and RCB studies was eliminated in 1976. But even had it continued and even had the studies produced a decisive effect on categorical health programs, this mode of rationalization could, at best, redirect resource

*Rationalisation des Choix Budgétaires.

allocation *within* the Ministry of Health. Because the ministry budget accounts for only 10 percent of total health expenditures, health planners both in the ministry and in the CGP all agreed that the challenge of rationalization was to control health expenditures by reducing excess capacity through the regulation of capital investment.

The legislative response to the call for rationalization came in 1970 with the enactment of the Hospital Law.[37] This legislation sought to control private sector growth and promote a "harmonious distribution" of health services. It called for reform of provider reimbursement methods to create financial incentives for the implementation of national and regional health plans. Above all, the Hospital Law aimed to improve management in the public sector and to contain the rate of growth (at public expense) of the private sector. To do this, new health planning and regulatory institutions were devised.[38] In 1973 a national commission was charged with producing a national health plan. Two regional commissions in each of France's 21 administrative regions were established to plan for health service needs and to authorize construction of new cliniques or extensions of existing ones in the private sector. The Hospital Law also divided the 21 regions into 284 health sectors. In each sector, public hospitals are required to provide a minimum range of services and to form cooperative unions (Groupement Interhospitalier—GIH) in which specialized personnel and medical technology can be shared. The private nonprofit sector is offered concessionary contracts by the GIH to assume responsibility for specific functions, take advantage of joint services, and thus become part of the so-called public hospital service.

At the national level, the health plan explicitly identified areas of need. In comparing present infrastructure levels to norms, health planners made public issues out of disparities. At the regional level, resource inventories were made for each of the 284 sectors. Norms were elaborated in terms of hospital bed population indices for specific medical disciplines; population projections were made for each region; and sometimes socioeconomic and epidemiologic characteristics of populations were taken into account in this process. The determination of norms was crude, but the work of the regional commissions is the largest effort, to date, to apply methods of health planning to the formation of health policy. Their plans—known as *cartes sanitaires* (health maps)—have become an essential document in the preparation of the national health plan and a critical tool in defining national health policy options.

The regional health planning commissions also bring together on a regular basis a wide range of leaders from the health sector. Representatives from public and private hospital associations, local government, regional and departmental health insurance funds, and physician and paramedical unions are obliged to meet and to confront issues of cost control, regionalization, and coordination. In this sense, health planning as rationalization introduces a different style of decision making for it extends health planning beyond the Ministry of Health to the arena of broad participation politics.

Implementation of the provisions of the Hospital Law has proceeded slowly. Cooperative unions of hospitals (GIHs) are not yet very cooperative. Though the regional health planning commissions have curbed duplication of hospital infrastructure by preventing the construction of some cliniques, they have not been given the authority to allocate health resources in the directions outlined by their plans. Although some nonprofit hospitals have joined the public hospital service, there have been no contracts bringing private cliniques into the system.[39] Although the total number of hospital beds is now considered sufficient, perhaps even excessive, health planning as rationalization has failed to reduce inequities in the distribution of hospital beds. Moreover, planners in the Ministry of Health, in the CGP, and particularly in the Finance Ministry, are alarmed by the continued growth of health care costs.

RUNAWAY COSTS AND STRATEGIES OF CONTROL

Between 1960 and 1980, the total consumption of medical services in France almost doubled from 4.0 to 7.5 percent of GDP (gross domestic product). That represents an average annual rate increase of 15 percent in current prices, and 7.5 percent, in 1970 constant prices.[40] Figures 4 and 5 depict secular trends—in current and in constant 1970 prices—of the average annual rate of increase for the three principal categories of medical care consumption: private hospitals, public hospitals, and ambulatory services in the private sector. Figure 6 depicts the average annual growth for aggregate medical consumption—public and private hospitals and ambulatory services combined—as well as for the expenditures of the CNAMTS.[41]

The purpose of figures 4 to 6 is merely to visualize long-cycle trends and to suggest what Lévy and others have already argued in depth: that the growth of health care costs in France reflects broad and complex processes of societal transformation.[42] An average annual rate of increase in health care consumption of 7.5 percent (in constant prices) over two decades is high (fig. 6). This point has been made time and again in the major reports on the problem of rising health care costs in France. What is noted less often is the secular decline in this growth rate from 1960 to 1980 (see fig. 6). Although, at first, this downward trend would suggest that the problem of rising costs is improving, a look at the secular decline of the GDP, in constant prices, over this same period, indicates that since 1973 the growth rate of the GDP has declined faster. This explains why rising health care costs continue to remain on the health policy agenda: they are felt even more strongly.

Since 1977, the economic situation has exacerbated the problem, because growing unemployment as well as slow economic growth have reduced the revenues of the NHI Funds thereby increasing their deficit.[43] What, then, can be done to balance the structural deficit in health care financing? In the crudest terms, health planners and policymakers

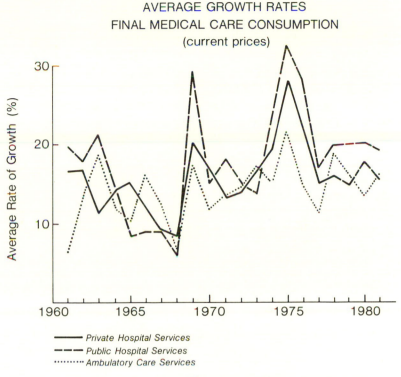

AVERAGE GROWTH RATES
FINAL MEDICAL CARE CONSUMPTION
(current prices)

Private Hospital Services
Public Hospital Services
Ambulatory Care Services

Fig. 4.

have two principal options: to increase revenues and to control expenditures.

METHODS TO INCREASE REVENUES

1. *Increase payroll taxes.* Payroll taxes for health insurance provided by the CNAMTS are currently equal to 18.95 percent of the taxable wage base. Employees pay 5.5 percent on their full wage; employers pay 8 percent on the full wage and 5.45 percent on the wage below a monthly ceiling of 7,080 Francs ($1,770). Over the past eight years, payroll taxes for employers as well as for employees have been raised on six occasions as part of financial salvage operations to balance the social security budget.

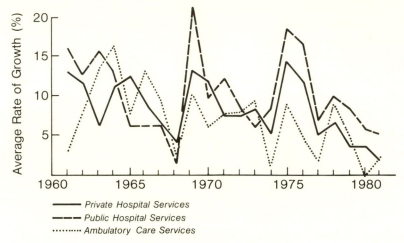

AVERAGE GROWTH RATES
FINAL MEDICAL CARE CONSUMPTION
(in 1970 constant prices)

——— *Private Hospital Services*
— — — *Public Hospital Services*
··········· *Ambulatory Care Services*

Fig. 5.

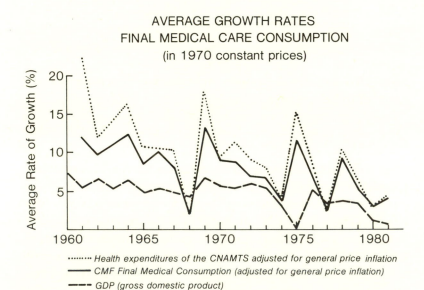

AVERAGE GROWTH RATES
FINAL MEDICAL CARE CONSUMPTION
(in 1970 constant prices)

··········· *Health expenditures of the CNAMTS adjusted for general price inflation*
——— *CMF Final Medical Consumption (adjusted for general price inflation)*
— — — *GDP (gross domestic product)*

Fig. 6.

2. *Raise wage ceilings.* To raise or even to eliminate the ceiling under which employer payroll taxes are assessed would increase revenues while simultaneously reducing inequalities since employers with employees earning wages above the current ceiling pay proportionately less than those with employees earning wages below the ceiling.

3. *Extend the taxable base.* Another method to raise health insurance revenues would be to tax capital in addition to labor or move toward a value-added tax. The main argument for a move in this direction is that the present tax burden penalizes labor-intensive industries and favors capital-intensive ones.[44] Moreover, during periods of recession the present mechanisms encourage employers to reward overtime work rather than increase the number of employees. One might, however, reasonably ask whether it makes sense to tax new investments when these are all the more necessary to restructure the present economy.

4. *"Fiscalize" the entire system.* Whereas raising the wage ceilings and extending the tax base represent methods by which to redistribute the tax burden of firms within the parafiscal system, financing social expenditures out of the government budget (through the fiscal system) is yet another option—one with very different economic and political implications.[45] Such a reform would eliminate the concept of contributory insurance schemes. Firms would be relieved of the tax burden they now bear but the state would be forced to increase taxes in order to finance the present level of social expenditures. Politically, this would shift power to the state and away from a corporatist social security organization managed by trade unions, and by the CNPF. The social security system would then fall under the public sector and be bound by its administrative procedures. Parliament would have to approve its annual budget, all health personnel including physicians would become civil servants, and the degree of administrative centralization would most likely increase.

5. *Increase private financing.* Roughly 80 percent of French health expenditures are collectively financed by the CNAMTS and the Ministry of Health. That leaves 20 percent in the form of private financing by individual out-of-pocket payments. One way to finance the growth of health expenditures is simply to increase the share of private financing through copayments or deductibles. This method would probably result in individuals subscribing to private health insurance to protect themselves against their increased risk.

METHODS TO REDUCE EXPENDITURES

1. *Price controls.* Regulation of prices, in France, is a well-established tradition and the health sector is no exception to the imposition of administrative pricing. On the demand side, policymakers can attempt to reduce utilization of services by raising the level of copayments and deductibles. On the supply side, policymakers can manipulate reimbursement rates for physicians in private practice as well as for private and public hospitals.

Demand-side policies are strictly limited in a society that has grown accustomed to NHI. Nevertheless, a number of minor measures can be taken whose effectiveness depends on the price elasticity of demand with respect to the service in question. In 1977, for example, the Council of Ministers reduced reimbursement rates for certain nonessential drugs from 70 to 40 percent of the controlled prices. In 1980, the government imposed a copayment as well as a deductible for long-term hospitalization: copayments above 80 Francs ($12) a month for 6 months or above a total of 480 Francs ($70) were thereafter assumed by the CNAMTS.[46]

On the supply side, regulation of physican fees is one of the cornerstones of French health policy. As we have seen, negotiations with the medical profession have resulted in agreement by a large majority of physicians to accept nationally set fees. The problem, however, is that the national fee schedule is more of an instrument for purposes of billing the NHI funds than an instrument for giving price signals to physicians so as to encourage them to behave in ways that are cost effective. Since the determination of physician fees is the result of negotiations between professional medical associations, the CNAMTS, and the government, it also reflects the relative power of medical specialty groups to negotiate advantageous fees for the procedures controlled by their disciplines.[47] In short, although negotiation of the fee schedule is a critical institutional mechanism for controlling reimbursement rates to physicians in private practice, it is not necessarily an effective instrument of price control.

In addition to physician reimbursement rates, French policymakers also control reimbursement rates to cliniques and to public hospitals. From the point of view of price control, however, coordination is exceedingly difficult to achieve because the CNAMTS negotiates the rate of the patient day for cliniques, whereas the department prefect, on instructions from the Ministry of Health as well as the Ministry of the Budget, sets the rate of the patient day for public hospitals.[48]

2. *Volume controls.* In an open-ended system characterized by fee-for-service payment under NHI, the problem with price controls is that the volume of services can often be adjusted to compensate for rigid price regulation. This is true for private practice in the ambulatory sector as well as for cliniques and public hospitals. As a result, health planners have also attempted to control the volume of services provided.

In the ambulatory care sector (since the collective contract of 1976) the system of statistical profiles on the procedures performed by each physician was computerized. The rationale has been to control the quality of medical care and to sensitize physicians to the financial implications of their activities. The system is based on finding irregularities in medical practice and issuing sanctions to doctors who overprescribe tests and drugs. This is exceedingly difficult, however, because criteria on proper workloads have not yet been agreed on. If the entire medical profession is influenced by reimbursement incentives to increase medical procedures, particularly specialty services and high-technology medicine, or if it is influenced by cultural norms to overprescribe drugs, the effect of the profiles will be negligible.

Since 1980, all French physicians receive periodic statements summarizing the consultations and procedures for which they have billed the CNAMTS through the intermediary of their patients. Enormous amounts of data have been collected on patterns of physician activity. Information is currently being collected by the CNAMTS on the sociodemographic characteristics of physician clientele populations. This is critical for it will one day enable the CNAMTS to go one step beyond pointing up disparities in the procedures performed by physicians; it will enable the CNAMTS to ignore disparities easily explained by such factors as age and sex and to investigate selectively the seemingly less justifiable disparities.

In the hospital sector there have been isolated attempts to control volume and regulate quality of care. There has been, however, no systematic effort comparable to the physician profiles either in the clinique or in the public hospitals. When volume controls have been imposed in the hospital sector, they have aimed largely at procedural issues to reinforce the price controls. For example, they have attempted to put limits on allowable rates of expenditure increase and to regulate administrative procedures such as hospital budget review.[49] Although French hospitals are not financed on the basis of closed budgets, estimated budgets may be inferred indirectly once one knows the allowable patient day rates and the estimated number of patient days.

With respect to cliniques, more refined classification schemes have been devised within which to regulate expenditure increases of like groups of institutions. As for public hospitals, every year a circular is issued by the Ministry of Health, after consultation with the Ministry of the Budget and the Ministry of Social Security (now part of the Ministry of Social Affairs) which sets the allowable rate of increase for all hospital budgets. In addition, entire categories of expenditure within hospitals have been strictly limited, and new positions for full-time staff have been denied by the Ministry of Health.[50]

3. *Capital controls.* In contrast to price controls and volume controls that are short-run methods to contain expenditures, capital controls are designed to contain long-run health expenditures. They aim to limit hospital expansion and modernization plans, capital expenditures for new medical technologies, and the production of new human capital, that is, doctors. Although controls on hospital investment have been a part of national economic planning in France since 1946, controls on the supply of medical manpower are relatively new.

As already noted, the Hospital Law of 1970 strengthened regulation of hospital facilities and capital expenditures. Over a period of ten years (1970–1980) the rejection rate on hospital investment requests (in the private sector) increased from 55 percent to over 80 percent.[51] As for the public sector, a series of new circulars as well as a new law have increased the Ministry of Health's authority over the growth of public sector hospitals.[52] In 1976 the government decided to stabilize the aggregate number of hospital beds in France. On December 29, 1979, the government passed a law granting the minister of health authority to close down hospital beds in the public sector.

Along with the law granting the minister of health power to close down hospital beds, the government passed legislation reducing the number of physicians trained by cutting enrollments in the medical schools. In effect, since 1971 the ministers of health and of education were granted the authority to control indirectly the supply of physicians by controlling entry into the medical school pipeline. The criteria for controlling entry were supposed to reflect the university's capacity for training physicians. In 1979, however, when it was declared that the number of medical students accepted into their second year of training would drop over a few years from 9,000 to 5,000, there was no longer any doubt about the fact that France had imposed a *numerus clausus.* One may speculate about the extent to which it will control long-run health care costs, enhance the prestige of the medical profession, or at least conserve its income.

THE POLITICS OF RATIONALIZATION

Health expenditures of the CNAMTS account for roughly one-third of total social security expenditures and 7.2 percent of the GDP. In addition to health expenditures, pensions and family allowances contribute to the vast income and expenditure flows that are administered by the social security system. Since 1971 the "social budget"—all state welfare expenditures and social security transfer payments—has exceeded the state budget as a whole;[53] and it currently equals over one-fourth of the French GDP.[54]

The Ministry of Finance has not ignored the growth of such expenditures and indirect taxes, for they increase fiscal and parafiscal pressures (from income and payroll taxes) and affect both disposable income and the production costs of industry. Increasing costs of production get passed on to consumers either through real wage losses or price increases, and this runs counter to the goal of the Ministry of Finance to promote industrial development and international competitiveness. Continued growth of health expenditures has forced consideration of two central economic questions for national health policy: (1) Should the rate of increase of the social budget be permitted to exceed the rate of increase of GDP? (2) Are the marginal benefits worth the rising costs to patients and taxpayers? The Finance Committee of the Sixth Plan answered both questions with a categorical no;[55] so did the 1976 economic plan of Prime Minister Raymond Barre.[56] And so has the present government of President Mitterand.

In spite of the widespread agreement on the need to contain health care costs, the two principal options for cost control—increasing revenues and containing expenditures—are politically difficult to implement. On the expenditure side, as noted in the preceding section, price controls, volume controls, and capital controls have been tried. They have not succeeded, however, in slowing the growth of health care costs. One reason is that all these strategies do not alter the way in which the health system is presently organized and financed.

On the revenue side, the most frequently proposed strategies to generate new funds for the health system have included financing the social security system out of the government budget, increasing health insurance premiums (payroll taxes), and raising the wage ceilings to which the payroll taxes are applied. Such measures provoke vigorous response, however.

The Finance Ministry wants to reduce government expenditures in order to have a more balanced budget. Employers resist increased payroll taxes, for such taxes increase wage costs, leading to higher production costs and prices, and thereby hurt their competitive position. Wage earners fight increased payroll taxes through trade unions; upper-level executives refuse to consider elimination of the wage ceilings; and special beneficiaries such as miners, merchant seamen, and railway workers do not merely oppose increasing payroll taxes but fight to protect their own particular and often advantageous insurance benefits. Beneficiaries of health insurance agree on only one point—that their premiums not be increased.

Despite these political pressure groups, policymakers have judiciously combined all these proposed stopgap measures to raise the revenues to finance rising health care costs. The result has been to leave the delicate balance between interest groups unaffected. Thus a political stalemate has emerged whereby short-term financial deficits are reduced while the basic structure of the French health system stays the same.

To change the health system in the directions laid out by health planners would require changing the financial incentives that influence provider behavior, increasing the Ministry of Health's authority over the allocation of health resources or at least coordinating its policies with those of the CNAMTS. There are both institutional and political obstacles, however, to implementing this remedy.

Since the CNAMTS finances the bulk of health services—roughly 70 percent of total health expenditures (see fig. 7) and 30 percent of the capital for hospital construction and modernization—its policies represent a strong lever for the implementation of national and regional health plans. But the CNAMTS is administratively separate from the Ministry of Health and has a political logic of its own. Despite the administrative reform of 1967, the social security system represents a political style most unlike the centralized and nonparticipatory politics of the Ministry of Health. It is one of those rare French administrative structures in which a tradition of accountability, decentralization, and regional autonomy is strong.[57]

In French administrative law, the CNAMTS is a private organization charged with the management of a public service. In reality, it is quasi-public. Its principal revenue-generating mechanism—payroll tax rates—must be approved by the Ministry of Social Security, which oversees the activities of the entire social security system. The eligibility and level of benefits of insurance coverage are determined by Parliament. Reimbursement policies for physicians and cliniques, however, are devised and negotiated by the CNAMTS board of directors. Since vast sums of money are involved, the government participates in the negotiations and oversees the entire process. Nevertheless, the CNAMTS is a strategic political force in health planning, particularly with regard to cost-control policies.

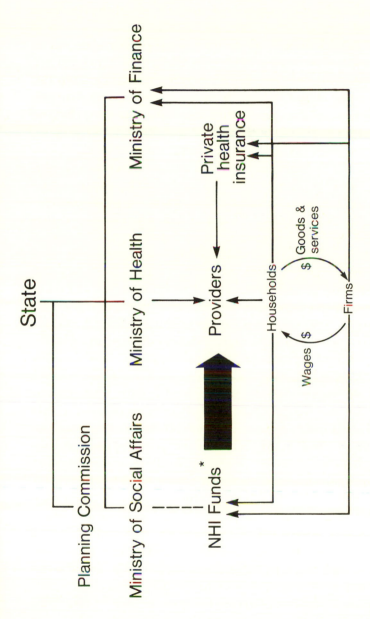

Fig. 7. Health Care Financing in France

*The principal NHI Fund is the *Caisse Nationale d'Assurance Maladie des Travailleurs Salariés* (CNAMTS)

Although the CNAMTS financially supports the entire health sector, it does not have jurisdiction over the determination of hospital-day rates in the public sector, and it negotiates with the private sector against powerful demands by hospital associations as well as the medical profession. For public hospitals, the per diem rate is officially set by the government. The CNAMTS merely pays the bill. For private cliniques, the per diem rate is negotiated by the CNAMTS. And for both public hospitals and cliniques, physicians' fees are also reimbursed.

If one were to design a model of a cost-maximizing health system, the French system would be a good first approximation of the kinds of provider reimbursement incentives one would want to include.[58] In the public and private sectors alike, French NHI provides powerful financial incentives for hospital managers to maintain high occupancy rates and to extend lengths of stay in order to increase revenues. There are no financial incentives for hospitals to develop large outpatient departments since they are reimbursed on the basis of costs incurred for their inpatient services. Nor are there incentives for hospitals to encourage ambulatory surgery, home care programs, and other less costly modes of health care delivery.

The incentives that influence health care providers in France are not the result of explicit policies democratically set and forcefully pursued by the CNAMTS. The board of directors of the CNAMTS has never pursued explicit policies such as hospital construction and modernization, or health-sector rationalization, let alone health promotion. Rather, the CNAMTS has responded to pressures emanating from the strongest recipients of its funds—the medical profession. When health planners in the Ministry of Health and in the CGP propose to rationalize the health sector by linking health plans to adjustments in provider-reimbursement rates, the medical profession and hospital associations emerge as a powerful barrier to change.

Rationalization of major resource-allocation decisions through health planning has provoked conflict throughout the health sector because of the effects of proposed reforms on different interest groups. This has exacerbated strains between planners and managers who seek to extend their control over the directions of health sector change by reorganizing the delivery system, and physicians and hospitals who fight to maintain their control and resist bureaucratic intrusion into their affairs. This conflict is real and the stakes are high for all concerned: the state, the medical profession, and the ancillary interest groups.

EVALUATION OF FRENCH HEALTH PLANNING

Three critical problems—all widely recognized by French health planners—have been periodically addressed, then quietly dismissed, and remain, to this day, unresolved. First, what constitutes an appropriate role for hospitals within the health system? Second, what responsibilities should be given to preventive medicine and public health? Third, what role should the principal payer play in health planning?

France was one of the first European countries to classify and eventually reorganize its hospitals in relation to the concept of regionalization.[59] The 1958 Hospital Reform Act envisaged the regional teaching hospital as the pivotal institution around which the health system functioned. In contrast, the task force on The Future of the Health System made a case for regionalization of health services so as to enable substitution of ambulatory community-based care for hospital care, whenever possible.[60] Recently, the Gallois-Taib Report criticized the lack of coordination between hospital services and la médecine libérale and urged the government to strengthen the organization of health services outside the hospital sector.[61]

In spite of the attention devoted to defining a proper role for the hospital, the administrative and organizational separation between hospital services and la médecine libérale remains a major obstacle to continuity in the French health care system. In addition, poor coordination often leads to excessive reliance on hospital care for services that would best be provided outside an institution. Under the present government, it appears that the Ministry of Health (under a communist minister) favors a hospital centered health system whereas the Ministry of Social Affairs (under a socialist minister) favors reinforcing the community-based ambulatory care sector.

As for the responsibilities of preventive medicine and public health, in March of 1982, minister of health, Jack Ralite designated four regions that will receive a starting budget with which to initiate a range of prevention programs. Assuming that these programs remain a political priority and that they are effective, it follows that they will reduce significantly the burden of disability and disease associated with alcoholism, smoking addiction, and poor working conditions. To increase their effectiveness, such programs in occupational health and safety, environmental control, and health education need to be supported by epidemiological research and evaluation, but this has traditionally been a weak area in France.

The problem of what role the principal payer for health services (CNAMTS) should play in health planning is especially controversial for the CNAMTS has no authority over the way in which hospitals manage the funds they receive under NHI. The CNAMTS is a powerful actor in the national fee negotiations with the medical profession as well as with other health professions. But these negotiations avoid explicit discussion of health policy issues such as redistribution of medical manpower between specialties or between geographic regions. In principle, negotiations over fee schedules are supposed to focus on the determination of reasonable fees based on relative costs. In practice, however, the resulting fees are determined neither by relative costs nor by health policy criteria but rather by skill in bargaining and by the relative power of medical specialty associations. For these reasons, the CNAMTS has been unable to reinforce the goals of health planners to rationalize the health sector.

Health planning as hospital construction and modernization succeeded because there was agreement on the goals and the Ministry of Health controlled the allocation of investment funds to hospitals. But health planning as rationalization appears to have failed because there are two conflicting goals—equity and cost containment—and neither the CGP nor the Ministry of Health controls the terms of provider reimbursement.

To date, despite efforts to rationalize the allocation of health resources, there are many problems. There are serious gaps between national and regional health plans and their implementation; the medical paradigm is still predominant; medical services are still heavily based in hospitals; primary care programs and health promotion are still marginal activities; and regionalization of services is still in the province of the health planner's dream. What is more, health care costs have continued to rise to the point that it hardly seems an exaggeration to suggest that French health planning is currently no more than a national strategy—or aspiration—to contain rising health care costs.

In summary, the CGP has presided over a process of formal health planning in which it has convened numerous commissions and special task forces. It has succeeded in forcing a wide range of health sector representatives to exchange views, in coordinating various state ministries, in sponsoring studies and assembling data on health sector trends, and in raising key issues and new ideas. The critical health policy decisions, however, have been taken outside the CGP. It has therefore not succeeded in redirecting the allocation of resources in the health sector.

What is most perplexing about French health planning is the attribution of responsibilities among central actors in the system. The CNAMTS finances health care expenditures without exercising management controls on what is provided; the central government, through the Ministry of Health, exercises a titular control over all public hospitals even though it finances only a small fraction of total health expenditures; and physicians determine the mix and quantity of resources used even though they share no financial responsibility, either in hospitals or in private practice.

Since the CNAMTS controls the purse strings, it sets implicit policies. These policies do not necessarily coincide with the goals of health planning. In fact, they often work at cross-purposes. For example, provider reimbursement incentives encourage the multiplication of medical procedures and of patient days spent in hospitals, whereas policymakers are concerned with controlling rising health care costs by shifting the burden of care from inpatient to outpatient services and fostering health promotion rather than high technology curative services.

Effective control of health costs depends on the state's ability to control the many factors that account for these mounting costs. In addition, it depends on the extent to which the state is able to link its explicit policies to the implicit incentives that govern provider reimbursement. Indeed, the problem of linking health planning to provider reimbursement has become a central issue in French health policy, one that is likely to determine whether health planning will succeed in influencing the allocation of health resources in the future.

6

HEALTH PLANNING AMID INSTITUTIONAL RENOVATION: QUEBEC

In Canada, there is neither a tradition of French-style national economic planning nor a formal process of national health planning. In contrast to the experience of the United States, there has been broad acceptance of a major governmental role in orienting the organization of health services. In the public health field, Canada is well known for the work of its Long-Range Health Planning Branch; in particular, for a report by the former minister of health and welfare, Marc Lalonde: *A New Perspective on the Health of Canadians*.[1]

The Lalonde Report is based on the notion that health problems must be analyzed in relation to four broad elements—human biology, environment, life-style, and health care organization. These elements, known in the Lalonde Report as a "health field concept," were identified by examining the epidemiology of sickness and death. The conclusion of the report stressed the importance of raising "human biology, environment and life-style to a level of categorical importance equal to that of health care organization, so that all our avenues of improved health are pursued with equal vigor."[2] This approach encouraged health planners to rank proposed health interventions on the basis of risk factor reduction and to place more emphasis on a range of prevention programs. Although the publication of the Lalonde Report in 1974 was a landmark in health planning, many of these ideas, as well as other innovative ones, were developed in the late sixties in Québec.

More than that of any other province of Canada, the government of Québec has aggressively intervened in the health sector to the point of encouraging planning efforts that would be inconceivable in other provinces.[3] Beginning in 1967, the Castonguay-Nepveu Commission developed a strategy for social change. Health planning served as an instrument for broadening the scope of medical care to include reform of welfare and social services. In 1970, the Ministry of Health embraced the health field concept and attempted to implement the recommendations of the Castonguay-Nepveu Commission. A vast program of legislative reform ensued; but as we shall see, the original proposals for social reform were quickly displaced by strategic objectives, and the pursuit of reform—although surely more far-reaching than elsewhere—was nevertheless compromised by political and economic constraints.

ORIGINS OF HEALTH PLANNING

Until 1970, the role of formal health planning in Québec was minimal. Following World War II, from 1945 to 1960, there was a period of great inertia. The economy was dominated by Anglo-Canadian and American industries that successfully exploited Québec's natural resources and cheap labor. The polity was dominated by the Union Nationale party under the leadership of Maurice Duplessis. And the church was the foremost institution of social control. Intervention by the provincial government in the economy was limited, and the health sector was left largely under the influence of the church and sometimes the marketplace.

In 1960 under the slogan "*Il faut que ça change*," the Liberal party succeeded in riding a wave of change. Indeed, during the decade between 1960 and 1970, Québec was entirely transformed. The role of religious institutions declined dramatically; the birthrate dropped from 30 per thousand population in 1950 to 28 in 1959 and 14.6 in 1972; provincial government expenditures increased by a factor of 32; and public sector employment increased from 36,000 in 1960 to slightly less than 350,000 in 1971.[4] The origins of health planning must be interpreted in the light of this so-called quiet revolution.

Although there was almost no public control over hospitals until 1970, the decade from 1960 to 1970 was one of rapid hospital growth and significant health sector transformation. As in France and the United States, this growth was fueled by large injections of government financing. In 1957, the federal government in Canada passed the Hospital Insurance and Diagnostic Services Act, which offered to finance roughly 50 percent of the cost of a provincial hospital insurance program. Faced with this irresistible offer of financial support, Québec passed the Hospital Insurance Act in 1961. Subsequently, in 1962, Québec passed the Hospitals Act requiring legislative authorization for all hospitals and administrative compliance with specified regulations. The effect of both of these legislative acts was to modernize hospital infrastructure and to initiate an era of increasing government concern with issues of hospital payment and planning.

In Québec, after the passage of hospital insurance, it became increasingly difficult for the religious orders to obtain charity donations and special government subsidies. After a brief period of reliance on the private money market and on government-backed bonds, the debts of religious hospitals were gradually taken over by the provincial government; and the hospitals became, in fact, public institutions, in spite of the private, nonprofit status of their governing boards. Spurred by insurance reimbursement incentives that favored hospital-centered medical care rather than less costly alternatives, public hospitals grew. By 1972 only 13 percent of hospitals in Québec belonged to religious orders, and their beds were mostly for psychiatric and long-term care.[5]

There were other changes in health care organization that accompanied the growth of public hospitals: health sector employment surged, and unionization of employees grew. Forty percent of the 100,000 new members in the confederation of trade unions worked in the health sector.[6] Even the medical profession became unionized. General practitioners and specialists formed two rival trade unions,* and the hospital association was strengthened. By the end of the 1960s, there were already strikes of health professionals in Montreal hospitals.

In 1965 the Canadian Parliament passed the Medical Care Act. The federal government offered to pay roughly 50 percent of the cost of health insurance for ambulatory medical care, providing that provincial governments do the following: (1) administer the insurance program on a non-profit basis, (2) provide comprehensive medical services, (3) provide universal coverage, and (4) allow coverage to be transferable from one province to another.

In 1966 the election of the Union Nationale government of Daniel Johnson delayed adoption of medical insurance in Québec for four years. This allowed some time for public debate over alternative models of health and social service delivery. Johnson appointed a Commission of Inquiry on Health and Social Welfare to study the health, welfare, and social service sectors and to propose desirable changes. This commission, under the direction of a highly reputed actuary, Claude Castonguay, allowed Johnson to delay acting on the federal Medical Care Act. In so doing, it initiated the first major health planning effort in Québec. The second major effort came four years later when Claude Castonguay

*Fédération des Médecins Omnipraticiens du Québec; Fédération des Médecins Spécialistes du Québec.

was named minister of health and attempted to implement the commission's recommendations.

HEALTH PLANNING AS A STRATEGY
FOR SOCIAL CHANGE:
THE CASTONGUAY-NEPVEU COMMISSION

The Castonguay-Nepveu Commission represented a major health planning effort both in its mandate and in the methods followed to fulfill it. The mandate was no less than to inquire into the entire health and social welfare field, identify problems, and recommend changes. The commission's methods of investigation involved establishing research committees; requesting detailed studies by specialists; soliciting briefs from agencies, associations, and individuals; and organizing public hearings. Thus, it combined three essential ingredients of exemplary public planning: analysis, design, and some participation by various groups in order to reach a consensus.

Since the commission began its work in the context of the medical insurance debate, the first volume of the report concerned this issue. Released in 1967, this report favored a universal health insurance plan for Québec.[7] Moving beyond such conventional therapy, however, the remaining volumes of the commission report, as well as Castonguay's speeches, contained unsparing criticisms of Québec's health system in general and physicians and Ministry of Health bureaucrats in particular. They criticized the absence of explicit health policies for Québec, the regional disparities in the distribution of morbidity and mortality and of health resources, the overemphasis on curative medicine, the negligence of community health, and the growth of health care costs.

The Castonguay-Nepveu Commission proposed an elaborate strategy for social change in Québec. In essence, it made a case for broadening the scope of medical care to include reform of welfare and social services. The strategy involved better planning, coordination, and administration of the entire health, welfare, and social services sectors in order to contain mounting costs and to reallocate health resources to improve health and not just the efficiency of medical institutions. Five ideas dominate the final, seven-volume report:[8]

Planning. The commission argued that the Ministry of Health should not merely administer categorical programs but should play a central role in health planning by assuming responsibility for resource allocation.

Regionalization. The commission argued that planning in the Ministry of Health should be regionalized and decentralized. It recommended that the province be divided into three regions. Each region would exercise control over financing for both capital and operating expenditures and delivery organizations such as hospitals would be responsible for the internal allocation of their budgeted resources.

A comprehensive approach to medicine. The commission criticized the traditional medical paradigm and advocated a new concept of health, *la médecine globale*, which stressed social and environmental factors of disease. It urged the development of a strong primary-care sector composed of general practitioners and social service workers and suggested that a multidisciplinary team of health professionals be given responsibility for the health of a designated population.

Participation. In order to broaden the context in which decisions concerning health resource allocation had traditionally been made, the commission suggested that all health planning and delivery organizations be required to institutionalize mechanisms for consumer and worker participation.

Reassessment of professional status. The commission proposed reducing inequalities between health sector professionals. It questioned existing criteria for licensing and certification and recommended distinguishing more carefully between organizations responsible for protecting the economic interests of the professions and those responsible for controlling the quality of professional practice.

Most noteworthy about the Castonguay-Nepveu Commission are the comprehensive solutions put forth to plan Québec's health system and to formulate an explicit health policy. The five key ideas outlined above indicate the broad directions in which the commission hoped to move the health sector. The effort to implement these ideas, beginning in 1970, reflects both the promise of and the obstacles to comprehensive health planning.

HEALTH PLANNING AS LEGISLATIVE REFORM

Phase I: The Castonguay Legacy

As the Castonguay-Nepveu Commission moved toward completion of its report, Castonguay decided to run for a seat in the National Assembly while Nepveu took over the chairmanship of the commission. Castonguay was elected in 1970 and promptly was appointed minister both of health and of family and social welfare. Backed by strong legislative support and a large part of the commission working with him in the ministry, Castonguay set out to turn the commission's plan into a reality. Among the measures adopted to revamp the health sector, one unilateral directive and five legislative bills are noteworthy for their bold aims and for the speed with which they were enacted:

1. *Hospital cuts.* Since the Castonguay Commission had indicated that an "excess supply" of hospital beds was

heavily concentrated in the acute sector, in May 1970, Castonguay issued a directive to sharply curtail hospital construction. Out of some 120 projects being planned or actually under construction and estimated to cost $498 million, 98 were suspended at a savings of $400 million, thereby saving many billions in future operating costs.[9] In addition, a large number of small, inadequate hospitals were closed, and efforts were made to convert short-term facilities to long-term care institutions and to consolidate obstetric and pediatric units.

2. *A new ministry.* In November 1970, Bill 42 was enacted, merging the Ministry of Health and the Ministry of the Family and Social Welfare into one Ministry of Social Affairs. The new ministry was no longer only to provide public health services and administer categorical programs. It was now responsible for social services as well as for the process of setting priorities, planning, programming, and evaluating.

With respect to the health sector, the Ministry of Social Affairs was organized to assure vigilant monitoring of hospitals and other health institutions (see fig. 8).[10] The largest department—financing—is in charge of forecasting the costs of all health and social service programs. It is also responsible for studying and approving budgets and controlling the reimbursement of operating as well as capital expenditures. The Planning and Programming departments are responsible for formal planning and implementation activities; but, as already indicated in this chapter, comparable activities were initiated prior to the creation of these departments. As we shall see, planning has continued in spite of a 1978 reorganization that eliminated the Planning Department. The major achievements of the Planning and Programming departments were to initiate systematic analyses of the population's health, social service, and income maintenance requirements; to design new programs; and, above all, to evaluate existing programs.

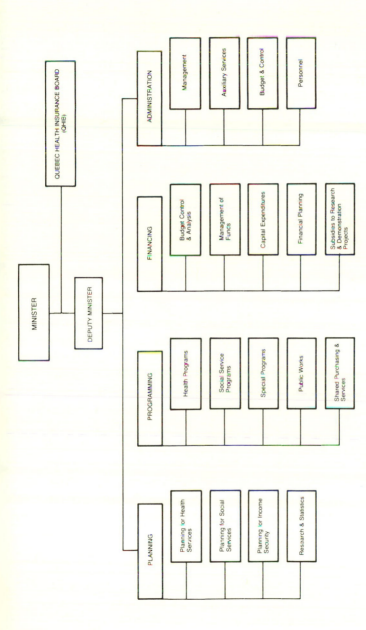

Fig. 8. The Ministry of Social Affairs: organization chart (1973)*

*The social welfare and income security departments have been omitted from this organization chart.

Source: Ministère des Affaires Sociales, Rapport Annuel 1973–1974 (Québec: Gouvernement du Québec, 1974)

The Professional Relations Department is responsible for negotiations with professional trade unions in the health sector. In addition, it serves in a consulting role to the ministry on matters of personnel administration and upgrading. Since personnel costs represent over 70 percent of hospital operating expenditures, the ability of this department to assist in relocating and retraining employees has been a critical component of Québec's cost control policy. Finally, the administrative department has developed a management information system for the ministry.[11] It has also assisted in improving administrative procedures, preparing the ministry budget, and supervising the population register.

3. *Health insurance.* In November 1970, Bill 8, the Health Insurance Act, was finally passed, establishing a system of universal medical insurance for the entire population of Québec. In addition to respecting the four conditions necessary to obtain federal assistance (see p. 120), this legislation explicitly protected clinical freedom, free choice of the doctor by the patient, and medical confidentiality. Bill 8 rejected the principle of a copayment and consequently made medical care in Québec free at the point of consumption.

From the perspective of providers, Québec NHI is innovative insofar as it does not limit physician reimbursement to fee-for-service payment. There is also the possibility of salary payment for physicians working in public health programs and health centers. Both forms of payment are negotiated between physician trade unions and the Ministry of Social Affairs. The administration of the NHI program, however, is the responsibility of the Québec Health Insurance Board (QHIB).

4. *New institutions.* In 1971, Bill 65, the Act Respecting Health Services and Social Services, was passed, calling for reorganization of most health and social welfare institutions. It affirmed that every Québec resident has

the right to receive adequate, continuous, and personal health services . . . allowing residents . . . to choose the professional or institution from whom or which he wishes to receive health services or social services.[12]

Above all, the bill attempted to design a new health and social service system for Québec by implementing the more politically feasible ideas of the Castonguay-Nepveu Commission. More specifically, the act created the local health and social service centers (CLSC), the Departments of Community Health (DSC), and, most important from the point of view of health planning, twelve Regional Councils for Health and Social Services (CRSSS).*

The concept of the CLSCs was visionary. These health centers were to provide a comprehensive approach to medicine by dispensing medical care combined with professional social services and public health programs tailor-made for each community. A typical CLSC, for example, has a staff doctor who not only makes diagnoses and prescribes medicine but also takes the time to talk about the family's general health and suggests preventive measures to ward off problems. Shortly after the passage of Bill 65, 250 CLSCs were planned to serve as points of entry into the health system. Each one was required to establish an administrative council to decide on its programs, and at least five of the twelve members were required to be actual users of the center. In contrast to the traditional approach to medical care, doctors were not in charge. Instead, they were to be part of a multidisciplinary team on an equal footing with nurses, social workers, psychologists, and dietitians—all collaborating to provide comprehensive patient care with an emphasis on prevention and health education.[13]

The establishment of the DSCs, although not as radical a step as the creation of the CLSCs, was, nevertheless, a bold

---

*Conseil Régional de la Santé et des Services Sociaux. Although the Castonguay-Nepveu Commission had planned only three regions, the government created twelve.

step in promoting public health. Although the DSC is located within a hospital, it has no patients, unlike other hospital departments. What is more, it has a separate, protected budget to avoid competition for funds from other hospital departments. The principal mission of the DSC is to study the health problems of its target population and to design and organize public health programs. For example, a DSC coordinates preventive health services in collaboration with the CLSCs in its region. It is also responsible for initiating epidemiologic studies and estimating regional health care needs. In one sense, the DSC is nothing more than a traditional public health department. In symbolic terms, however, its insertion within the hospital expressed a new concern about community problems. When properly functioning, a DSC was supposed to stimulate other hospital departments to initiate preventive health services and eventually to coordinate them.

Finally, the creation of regional councils was perhaps the most far-reaching reform of Bill 65. These new institutions were responsible for organizing the participation of the population in defining its needs and in administering its health and social welfare institutions. In this sense, the regional councils are responsible for formal health planning. In addition, they advise and assist individual health care facilities in the design of their programs; they link the public, the Ministry of Social Affairs, and health and social service institutions; and they handle complaints about all facilities in their region.

During the first phase of health planning as legislative reform, the regional councils had limited regulatory authority and budgetary responsibilities. Their principal role lay in devising strategies for eliminating duplication of costly services and in promoting common support services between hospitals in the context of regional health plans. During the second phase, however, as we will see, pressure grew to rationalize the health sector, and the regional councils were granted more authority and were called upon to perform new administrative functions.

5. *New controls on the professions.* In July 1973, while the regulations for Bill 65 were being drafted, Bill 250, the Professional Code, was passed. This legislation restructured and standardized *all* licensed and certified occupations, not just those within the health sector. In addition, it created a new institution for controlling the quality of professional practice: the Québec Professions Board.* The aim of this reform was to protect the public served by the professions, including the medical profession. Thus, each professional corporation—for example, the Order of Physicians—was required to have one-half of its board of directors consist of consumer representatives chosen by the Québec Professions Board.

Needless to say, the above legislative reforms did not entirely coincide with all the recommendations of the Castonguay-Nepveu Commission. Many of the commission's ideas were far less practical than the planners had imagined. For example, the commission had advocated payment mechanisms other than fee-for-service; but once Castonguay became minister of social affairs, it became apparent, given the political constraints and the speed with which he wished to pass Bill 8, that fee-for-service was the only basis on which the medical profession would negotiate its predominant mode of reimbursement. In addition, despite the commission's original intention to create three powerful regions, Castonguay found the provincial government reluctant to relinquish central control and proceeded with a watered down regionalization plan that delegated virtually no power to the regional councils. Finally, despite the commission's emphasis on the social context of health, such broad goals were not readily accepted; and in the

*Office des Professions du Québec.

course of implementing the legislative reforms, they were
displaced by seemingly less important objectives.

Castonguay himself conceded in retrospect,

> We really believed that if we created a whole new set of objec-
> tives for health care and a brand new framework . . . all those
> working in the health field—doctors, nurses, and administra-
> tors—would get a new lease on life. . . . We hoped they would
> think in terms of prevention, education, rehabilitation and
> general improvement in the health of the population; and our
> greatest aspiration was that they would work together as teams
> to achieve these goals. We now realize that this was a false
> expectation; we overestimated people's reactions; no one was
> really enamoured with the notion of new objectives.[14]

Beyond suffering from "false expectations," the commission found that once its objectives were translated into legislation, the reforms provoked vigorous response from the
medical profession. The Health Insurance Act produced
the greatest political conflagration. Since the plan was first
proposed by the commission in 1967, it had presented the
government with two central problems:

> In giving in to federally imposed conditions, Québec's
> decision to pass the Health Insurance Act represented a
> retreat from its evolution toward a more independent
> role in Canada.

> In releasing new expenditures for medical care, health
> insurance raised the specter of fiscal strain on Québec's
> economy, which was already suffering from a limited tax
> base and high tax rates.

When Castonguay resisted allowing more than 3 percent
of the physicians in a given specialty and in each of Québec's
administrative regions to opt out of the insurance plan, a
major struggle ensued.[15] The Québec Federation of Medical Specialists called a strike. The strike turned into a crisis,
but a back-to-work order issued to society's most prestigious

elite confirmed that the Québec government was prepared to implement the legislation and pursue health care reform.

PHASE II: THE PURSUIT OF REFORM

In 1973, Castonguay decided not to run for a second term in the National Assembly. The process of health care reform did not subside, however. Claude Forget succeeded Castonguay as minister of social affairs. Then in 1976, the Parti Québécois came to power, creating a political climate supporting independence from Canada and further social reform. During this post-Castonguay era, health planners and policymakers continued to promote new legislative reforms as well as to enforce and extend the Castonguay reforms. Above all, they sought to tighten control and reduce the fat in the hospital sector, to allocate government funds to other priorities, and to develop primary health care and social services. Concurrently, policymakers granted more power to the regional councils to promote decentralization. The result of those policies has led to implementation of a significant portion of the Castonguay plan for health care reform. In addition, it has crystallized health planning issues in Québec and thereby focused some attention on the problems of planning.

THE HOSPITAL SQUEEZE

Following Castonguay's suspension of major hospital construction programs in May 1970, the new administration of the Ministry of Social Affairs attempted to devise a method of hospital reimbursement that would effectively contain rising health care costs in the short run. In 1971 a payment method consisting of prospectively set annual budget limits—so-called global budgets—was introduced as a demonstration project in twenty-three hospitals.[16] In 1972 the global budget was gradually extended to the entire network of health and social service facilities.

Since the Ministry of Social Affairs finances the operating expenditures of Québec's hospitals, its plan was to establish a limit on the total amount that hospitals were allowed to spend. Hospital administrators, however, adopted the global budget with the expectation that they would maintain the discretion to manage hospitals as before and that the ministry would continue to cover any potential deficits just as it had in the past. During the first few years of global budgeting in Québec, expectations of the hospital administrators were correct. Hospital costs continued to increase at roughly the same rate as in the late sixties. Moreover, Québec's hospitals had become more expensive than those of richer provinces, and these differentials persisted under global budgeting, narrowing slightly between Québec and Ontario and increasing between Québec and Alberta (table 9).[17]

In an effort to change this trend, in 1974 during the first year of the Forget administration, the ministry announced that it would no longer pay the costs of deficits in operating expenditures of hospitals. Since there would be, in effect, no more end-of-the-year settlements to balance hospital budgets, the hospitals became part of a complex system of top-down government budgeting. Roughly 70 percent of hospital costs are attributed to personnel. Thus, the Québec government began the process of budget setting for hospitals by negotiating salaries, fringe benefits, and working conditions with provincewide hospital trade unions. As for the balance of the institutional budget—the nonlabor component of hospital costs—it was progressively reduced.

Since 1974, with few exceptions, if a hospital exhibited a deficit at the end of a year, before receiving its budget for the following year, it was responsible for presenting a retrenchment plan to financial officers at the ministry.[18] Where a budget surplus existed, there were two possible incentive payments. If the hospital successfully met the ministry's budget reduction objective it could keep 50 percent of the surplus, but the following year the budget base was reduced accordingly. If the hospital merely stayed

TABLE 9
AVERAGE COSTS PER PATIENT-DAY,
ALL ACUTE AND CHRONIC HOSPITALS

| | Dollars per patient-day | | | Ratio of Québec to | |
	Québec	Ontario	Alberta	Ontario	Alberta
1966	49.23	36.67	34.29	134.3	143.6
1967	55.60	43.12	39.58	128.9	140.5
1968	60.99	50.22	43.00	121.4	141.8
1969	71.31	54.51	47.22	130.8	151.0
1970	77.04	61.10	51.15	126.1	150.6
1971	85.00	68.10	55.25	124.8	153.8
1972	100.29	76.70	60.56	130.8	165.6
1973	105.45	83.03	64.38	127.0	163.8

Sources: J. Lefort, *Performances des hôpitaux: données comparatives de coût de l'hospitalisation et de l'efficacité des ressources au Québec, en Ontario et en Alberta—1966–1972, 1973 préliminaire* (Québec: Planification financière, Direction générale du financement, Ministère des Affaires Sociales, 1974), p. 45. Cited in W. Glaser, *Paying the Hospital in Canada* (New York: Columbia University, Center for the Social Sciences, 1980), p. VI-15.

under its authorized budget, it was free to use 10 percent of the surplus for any purpose.

Despite the negative sanction of presenting a retrenchment plan in the case of deficits and the positive incentives for staying within prescribed global budgets, the principle of inciting hospitals to save money at one point in time was ineffective because it resulted in the permanent reduction of the hospital budget base. Thus, many hospitals continued to run deficits and to present retrenchment plans to the Ministry of Social Affairs. At the end of the year, special bargains were struck between ailing hospitals and the ministry. In 1976, however, the economy was in such poor shape that the government imposed budget cuts on all acute hospitals by limiting their budget increase to a flat 2.5 percent.[19] In addition, to reduce long-run costs, a ministerial directive ordered all acute-care hospitals of 200 beds or more to convert at least 10 percent of their beds to chronic care.[20] This bold but impulsive policy highlighted the central problem of global budgeting for hospitals: how to ascertain their relative efficiency and thereby distinguish between those with excessive and those with insufficient budgets.

The methodological response to this problem came in 1976 with the development of a new method for setting prospective hospital budgets—budgetary base review (*révision de la base budgétaire*). The method involves grouping hospitals on the basis of their diagnostic case mix and comparing their relative costs.[21] The more efficient hospitals are those whose costs for similar activities are below its group's average. The less efficient hospitals are those whose costs for similar activities exceed its group's average. Beginning in 1977, budgetary base review was the principal criterion used in deciding how to allocate the yearly increment among hospitals and how to negotiate end-of-year settlements to promote efficient performance within the industry.

Whether the combination of global budgets and budgetary base review in Québec has increased hospital efficiency is impossible to say. Unfortunately, there has been no rigorous study of the effects of Québec's global budgets on the provision of hospital services. What we know is that hospitals have systematically received less than they have requested. For example, during the 1977–1978 fiscal year, they requested a 3.2 percent increase and got 0.7 percent; during 1980–1981, they asked for 10.9 percent and got 5 percent.[22]

In addition to trimming hospital budgets, the Ministry of Social Affairs, in collaboration with the universities and the Corporation of Physicians, has reduced the number of medical students, particularly those training to be specialists. As a consequence of such measures, hospitals have been forced to reduce expenditures through service reductions or adjustments in service mix and through more aggressive purchasing and consolidation of services. A McKinsey Company study indicates that between 1974 and 1976, there was virtually no growth of real per capita nonlabor costs in Québec hospitals.[23] William Glaser reports four major hospital responses to global budgeting: (1) changes in hospital

decision making so that competing claims on limited resources are now reviewed and resolved more explicitly; (2)
increasing acceptance of service consolidations; (3) a renewed growth of philanthropy and private development;
and (4) an attempt by hospitals to shift expenses from the
global budget base to its outpatient service, which can bill
the QHIB separately, thus adjusting for increases in service
intensity.[24]

Whatever its broader repercussions in the long run and
its more detailed short-term effects on the configuration of
hospital services, the imposition of prospectively set budget
limits in Québec has succeeded in squeezing the hospital
sector.

PRIORITIES

The hospital squeeze was not merely the work of tough-
minded financial controllers at the Ministry of Social Affairs; it was part of the Castonguay-Nepveu Commission's
overall strategy for health care reform. In 1976 a five-year
development plan for health care resources recapitulated
the main ideas of the Castonguay-Nepveu Commission.[25] It
analyzed the distribution of hospital and ambulatory services within the province and provided guidelines for
reducing the hospital sector and substituting new organizational modes of health care delivery, such as home care,
community nursing services, and CLSCs, for the increasing
proportion of the elderly, the handicapped, and the mentally ill in the population.

In contrast to the comprehensive recommendations of
the Castonguay Commission, the new development plan
explicitly identified criteria for resource allocation and proposed quantitative standards. For example, it recommended reducing the number of hospital beds from 4.8 to
3.2 per thousand population and urged prevention programs such as reduction of highway speed limits and man-
datory use of seat belts for car passengers, which was estimated to result in an annual reduction of 50,000 hospital

days per year.²⁶ In addition, the development plan analyzed regional disparities in the distribution of health resources, adjusted for interregional population flows, and identified priority regions in the north for resource investment: l'Outaouais, Côte-Nord, and Trois-Rivières.

Two years after the publication of the five-year development plan, a second important document was released by the Division of Planning at the Ministry of Social Affairs: *Guidelines for the Allocation of Specialized Resources.*²⁷ Based on a literature review of state-of-the-art medical opinion and practice, this document recommended criteria for resource allocation in the following specialties: surgery, including ambulatory surgery programs; intensive care; renal dialysis; computerized axial tomography (CT scanners); radiation therapy; and nuclear medicine. Although they were most useful from the point of view of provincewide health planning, by the time these guidelines were developed, formal planning criteria were considered of minor importance. Shortly after the publication of the health resource development plan, the Parti Québécois came to power, and the task of planning as legislative reform was resumed by the new minister of social affairs, Denis Lazure.

Beginning in 1976, Lazure focused on improving social services for juvenile delinquents, the physically disabled, and the elderly. In 1977, Bill 24, Protection of Youth, was passed to safeguard the rights of the young, increase youth programs, and thereby require the social services sector to assume some of the responsibilities previously assumed by the criminal justice system. In 1978, Bill 8, Rights of the Physically Disabled, was passed, creating the Office for the Disabled, charged with the task of coordinating services and promoting their integration both in schools and at work. As for the elderly, the ministry's budget for home help, home care, and community nursing programs doubled between 1977 and 1980.²⁸

In addition to new services for juvenile delinquents, the physically disabled, and the elderly, the new administration at the Ministry of Social Affairs promoted child care programs and occupational health. Bill 77, Child Care Services, created the Office for Child Care Services to assess needs, coordinate existing services, and subsidize the development of new services as well as the parental contribution of low-income people. Bill 17, Health and Work Safety, made occupational health the responsibility of the public health system.[29] It created the Commission on Health and Work Safety with equal representation of trade unions and employers and endowed it with significant regulatory power. It also created a network of health and work safety committees whose function is to hire physician specialists in occupational health, to enforce work safety regulations, and to analyze occupational health hazards of each of their regions. The significant innovation in this system is that occupational health physicians are no longer paid by the employers; they are paid out of public funds managed by regional health and work safety committees.

In light of these legislative reforms and of the clearly articulated policy to clamp down on hospitals in order to use the marginal savings to promote primary care and social services, it is striking to note the relative neglect of CLSCs during this phase of health care reform. In all the rhetoric of the Parti Québécois about independence and the need for rapid social change, there was never a clear position in favor of encouraging the growth of these local health centers. During the summer of 1977, Lazure told the press he would "meditate" on the subject during his vacation.[30] In 1978, the prime minister, René Lévesque, called for a "deep reevaluation" of CLSCs.[31] A year earlier, however, the federation of CLSCs of Québec had already evaluated itself and had shown that out of all general practitioners in Québec only 3 percent worked in CLSCs. Moreover, a survey of sixty out of a total of seventy-two CLSCs existing in 1976 indicated that there appeared to be more emphasis on the delivery of medical care than on psychosocial services and programs related to community action, youth, the elderly, and the physically disabled.[32]

Above all, the main complaint emanating from the federation of CLSCs was that the ministry had failed to link its social policies to the existing network of CLSCs. For example, with respect to occupational health, instead of enlarging the role of CLSCs, new institutions were created. With respect to juveniles, the CLSCs might have been asked to organize local youth groups and establish sports activities, but once again they were excluded. Finally, with respect to services for the physically disabled and the elderly, CLSCs might have benefited from an overall budget increase along with incentives to design innovative programs in these areas. Instead, the new funds went to social service centers (CSS),* new nursing homes, and new specialized programs.

CLSCs, particularly newly created ones, were encouraged to provide services within the ministry's priority areas. In particular, they were asked to organize home care services, solicit voluntary help, and provide health care to low income as well as geographically isolated groups. This was a far cry, however, from their original mission to link comprehensive health care to preventive services and community action programs and to become the point of entry to the health care system. Lazure stated explicitly that the CLSCs would do well to "reject the old dream of wanting to serve as the universal entry gate to health services."[33] Rather, he viewed their role as one of assuring complementary services to those of mainstream medical care.

It would be misleading to interpret the neglect of CLSCs as an accurate reflection of the priorities of the Parti Québécois. Having come to power in a period of general interest in cost containment strategies for health care, the government was naturally interested in promoting relatively inexpensive, community-based services that could substitute for more costly conventional hospital and ambulatory care. But as Frédéric Lesemann argues in his sociopolitical study of the stakes involved in Québec's health care reforms, the resistance of the medical profession and its powerful lobby at the Ministry of Social Affairs severely

*Centre de Services Sociaux.

constrained the avenues of feasible reform.[34] In this sense, it would seem more reasonable to interpret the neglect of CLSCs as a concession to the barriers to institutional change and to the problems of planning for health care reorganization in a predominantly fee-for-service health system with universal coverage under NHI.

PROBLEMS OF PLANNING AND THE REGIONAL COUNCILS

Despite the five-year development plan for health resources and the ministry's guidelines for the allocation of specialized resources, the patterns of reallocation called for in these documents have not been achieved. The problems concern not merely the organization of ambulatory care but hospitals as well.

With regard to ambulatory care, the fundamental problem has been the familiar one of failing to adjust provider reimbursement rates to encourage comprehensive primary-care services in CLSCs and discourage costly services in hospital outpatient departments, emergency rooms, and specialty polyclinics. Analysis of physician-induced expenditures in Québec suggests that physicians, by their decisions either to refer their patients or to provide diagnostic and therapeutic services, are responsible for the major portion of health care costs.[35] Moreover, studies of physician responsiveness to reimbursement incentives in Québec indicate that physicians tend to adjust the mix of their clinical procedures to maximize their earnings.[36]

The classic example of such conventional economic behavior in Québec is the case of reimbursement for the injection of varicose veins. In 1974 the QHIB reduced significantly the reimbursement rate for this procedure. In 1976 it sponsored a study that announced the following:

1. The QHIB's expenditures for the injection of varicose veins decreased by a factor of 26.5 percent in 1975.

2. The minor providers of the procedure (less than 9,000 injections per year) decreased their activity in 1975.
3. The major providers of the procedure increased their volume of procedures in an attempt to compensate for the reduction in reimbursement rate.[37]

In Québec, as in France, the fee-for-service mode of physician reimbursement tends to encourage technical procedures such as electrocardiograms and X rays. Time devoted to patient contact and to the intellectual component of differential diagnosis is not encouraged in comparison to the technical dimensions of medical practice. Whereas in France the National Health Insurance Fund (CNAMTS) is in many ways separate from the Ministry of Health, in Québec the Health Insurance Board is more effectively linked to the Ministry of Social Affairs. This has resulted in tougher bargaining between the government and the health professions. For example, in Québec, twenty-six routine diagnostic and therapeutic procedures cannot be billed separately to supplement a consultation. Further, there is a trimester income limit beyond which general practitioners receive only one-fourth of the normal reimbursement rate for billable procedures. In addition, physicians working in CLSCs and DSCs, as well as a small fraction of hospital-based physicians, are remunerated on a salaried basis by the QHIB.

In spite of these measures, provider reimbursement in Québec remains predominantly based on fee-for-service payment. A recent task force report on the remuneration of health professions in Québec criticizes the "pseudo-productivity" resulting from fee-for-service incentives and evokes the inherent conflict of interest between the clinical freedom of physicians to prescribe appropriate procedures and fee-for-service reimbursement for their services.[38] What is more, this report recognizes the failure of Québec policymakers to link planning goals to reimbursement incentives:

The system of fee-for-service payment does not function in an integrated way with the broader health system. In the first place a negotiating process serves as a substitute for planning and management; the objectives of negotiation have taken the form of rate-setting objectives or payment levels and they have hardly or not at all embraced the general objectives of planning for health care services.[39]

In light of the nature of reimbursement mechanisms in Québec, it would be surprising, indeed, if the patterns of ambulatory care sought by planners were achieved. As far as the hospital sector is concerned, the experience of planning must be judged a success to some extent. From the perspective of cost control policy, between 1976 and 1980 per capita health expenditures as a percentage of GDP stabilized (they decreased from 7.5 to 7.2).[40] These figures, no doubt, reflect the decrease in acute hospital beds (from 5.2 per 1,000 population in 1974 to 4.3 in 1977).[41] From the perspective of implementing planning guidelines and reallocating health resources both among and within geographic regions, however, new problems appear to be emerging. They are related to the recent efforts of the provincial government to decentralize administrative decision making.[42]

Since 1975 the role of the regional councils has evolved from an advisory body to one invested with authority. In April 1975 the Ministry of Social Affairs empowered the regional councils to authorize or deny all investments under $50,000 that were proposed by hospitals as well as by health and social service facilities. A year later, this policy was applied to all investments under $1,000,000. In addition, the regional councils were asked to make recommendations concerning all personnel hirings. In 1977, with the passage of Bill 10, important modifications were made to Bill 65, which originally established the regional councils. Bill 10 devolved some power from the Ministry of Social Affairs to the regional councils as well as to individual health facilities. Regional councils were henceforth entitled to establish new health facilities in their regions and to create administrative commissions composed of representative regional interests in the health sector. Individual health institutions were required to conform to the objectives elaborated by these bodies as well as to prepare their own internal plans.

In 1978, in an effort to decentralize the powers of the ministry, Bill 103 was passed to amend, once again, Bill 65 and enlarge the powers of the regional councils. By 1979, within each of the twelve regions, the regional council (CRSSS) was exercising four critical functions:

1. *Regional planning.* The CRSSS is responsible for establishing regional priorities and assessing health care needs. In addition, it must elaborate implementation plans that translate the ministry's health policies into a set of local initiatives.

2. *Programming.* The CRSSS is responsible for coordinating activities between hospitals and other health institutions such as CLSCs and social welfare agencies. If regional plans call for reallocation of health resources within a region, the CRSSS must program resources accordingly for review by the Ministry of Social Affairs.

3. *Financing.* Within a regional capital budget, the CRSSS is responsible for the distribution of funds among hospitals and other health and social service institutions.

4. *Control and evaluation.* The CRSSS is responsible for budget reviews of hospitals and other health and welfare institutions in the region. In addition, it must collaborate with the Ministry of Social Affairs to collect and analyze relevant data for purposes of evaluation and quality control.

In spite of having assigned the CRSSS the above functions, which are elaborated in a recent government document on decentralization,[43] the Ministry of Social Affairs has reserved for itself the final responsibility for the strategic allocation decisions: the determination of operating budgets for individual hospitals as well as other health service institutions and the distribution of investment budgets not merely among but also within regions. With regard to the determination of hospital budgets—for operating expenditures as well as for investments—since 1980, the ministry has, with few exceptions, followed the recommendations of the regional councils. This new process for making allocation decisions is likely, however, to raise new problems in the future.

What will happen to the budgetary base review method of setting global operating budgets for hospitals? Will the regional councils adopt this centrally defined method to encourage hospital efficiency on the basis of comparisons of similar institutions throughout Québec, or will other criteria, such as proposed norms or priorities specific to particular regions, emerge to guide the process of resource allocation? If new regional criteria emerge to promote intraregional equity or merely to salvage a region's most prestigious hospital, conflict will undoubtedly grow between the region and the center. If centrally proposed criteria are followed to the letter, then decentralization will be no more than an administrative exercise.

However this issue is resolved in Québec, the problem of deciding what criteria should guide the allocation of health resources is now, at last, widely acknowledged.[44] The challenge that remains is how to link agreed-upon decision-making criteria to the reimbursement incentives of the QHIB. For example, once a CRSSS agrees on its priorities, how can the allocation of hospital budgets and physician reimbursement incentives serve to implement health planning goals?

EVALUATION OF HEALTH PLANNING IN QUEBEC

It is exceedingly difficult and perhaps even misleading to evaluate health planning efforts in a system that has changed as rapidly as that in Québec. Marc Renaud argues that the social changes that occurred during the "quiet revolution," combined with the lack of managerial employment opportunities for Québécers in the Anglo-controlled private sector, led a "new middle class" to seek "social hegemony" in the provincial government.[45] In light of this argument, it is not surprising that the Castonguay-Nepveu Commission proposed far-reaching reforms and greater government intervention in the health sector or that the combination of health planning and rapid reform succeeded in reorganizing the Québec health system. But were health resources actually reallocated?

Writing in 1974, Jacques Benjamin criticized economic planning in Québec in the following terms:

> Everything that has been undertaken in the last twelve years in the field of planning only has an emotive value. . . . For the last twelve years, we have been working backward. We have consciously put the emphasis on the concept of planning while it would have been more fruitful to pay attention to the instruments; the fever from France has invaded the offices of the first planners. We wanted to apply the French model integrally to Québec, while Québec did not even possess some of the instruments enabling it to operationalize its plans, especially in the control of the economy, the coordination between state departments and even political stability in 1968–1970.[46]

Health planning as a strategy for social change in Québec produced a monumental blueprint of what the future health sector should look like. Health planning as legislative reform succeeded in implementing a considerable portion of the blueprint. Just as the planners failed to achieve "control" over the economy, however, they were also unable to control the health sector. As Renaud aptly concluded:

> The net results of these reforms were huge reorganizations and administrative reshufflings that, in a sense, did rationalize the allocation of resources. But, above all, these reforms seem either to have maintained or reinforced the powers or privileges of various categories of Francophone professionals, or to have created new interesting jobs for university-trained individuals in the state bureaucracy.[47]

As we have seen, the experience of the CLSCs supports the thesis that health planners were unable to achieve control over the health sector. Although the CLSCs represent one of the most innovative experiments in community health throughout the world, they have been beset by organizational problems since their inception. To begin with, the institutional boundaries of CLSCs were not clearly defined by Bill 65. As a result, they often ran into conflicts with the DSCs and the traditional CSSs. In addition, there developed a divergence among CLSCs. Some were service oriented, particularly in rural areas, that is, they concentrated on delivering health and social services; others were community oriented, that is, they concentrated on local political issues that they considered, along with Rudolf Virchow, "medicine on a large scale." For example, community-oriented CLSCs turned their attention to issues of poverty, occupational health, and pollution and often embarrassed the provincial government, including the Ministry of Social Affairs that financed them. Such activities did not usually increase the size of their budget allocations.

The service-oriented CLSCs provoked a strong response from the Québec Federation of General Practitioners. In order to counterbalance the competition of CLSCs, it organized the creation of roughly 450 polyclinics in which physicians are sovereign and are reimbursed on a fee-for-service basis by the QHIB.[48] The polyclinics range from small group practice offices to large multispecialty organizations. Often, their distinguishing characteristic is the quality of their twenty-four-hour reception services.

One might argue that the CLSCs were successful insofar as they were responsible for the proliferation of polyclinics, which certainly altered and probably even improved the nature of medical practice. The bulk of ambulatory care in Québec, however, is still provided largely in solo practice, polyclinics, or outpatient hospital departments. Although many of the CLSCs have made remarkable improvements in the direct provision of primary health care and social services to various communities that were poorly served

previously, they have thus far failed to significantly reallocate health resources toward comprehensive medicine.

The experience of health insurance in Québec also supports the thesis that health planners failed to control the
health sector. Enterline, McDonald, and their colleagues
have shown that health insurance succeeded in making
medical services more accessible to lower socioeconomic
groups.[49] As we have seen in relation to the problems of
planning, however, health insurance has so far failed to
serve as a financial lever to reallocate health resources.
Rather than serving to promote the reforms created by
Bill 65, the financial incentives built into the fee schedule,
combined with the predominant fee-for-service method of
physician reimbursement, have promoted the multiplication of medical procedures both within and outside hospitals.[50] Thus, health insurance has worked at cross-purposes
with the health planners' goals of shifting the burden of
primary care out of the hospitals and out of private practice
to the CLSCs.

Aside from the failure of planners to achieve control over
resource allocation in the health sector, the new structures
created by the legislative reforms, including the new professional code, have so far been unable to change the habits
and attitudes of both consumers and health professionals.
With the minor exception of a new group of specialists in
community health and, more recently, occupational health,
the health system is still largely dominated by physicians and
centered in hospitals and private practice. Since the Lalonde
Report at the federal level, ideas about prevention strategies
and public health priorities have been revitalized; but significant resources have not yet been invested in this
direction.

Nevertheless, these criticisms may well be premature,
given the rapid pace of change in Québec, for there are
some signs that health planning in the future might have
more impact on health resource allocation. A recent report
of a task force on the remuneration of health professionals
proposed radical reform of the reimbursement system:[51]

elimination of fee-for-service payment and the creation of a modular hourly payment system (*système des honoraires modulés*) based on time and expertise as determined by local physician committees charged with allocating global district budgets. Within this system, each professional would be paid on the basis of explicitly allocated tasks performed, ranging from health education and public health services to the provision of hospital and ambulatory medical services.

In addition, efforts to promote decentralization continue to grow stronger. The regional councils continue to be granted greater authority and more funds to plan and control the allocation of health resources within Québec's twelve health regions. The extent to which health planners will continue to be inspired by the ideas laid out in the Castonguay-Nepveu Report is uncertain. The extent to which policy will be guided more by regional planning criteria than by central ministry criteria will remain a major point of controversy. But whatever criteria dominate, there seems little doubt that the future of health planning in Québec depends largely on the power and capability of the regional councils to reallocate health resources.

7

HEALTH PLANNING IN A
NATIONAL HEALTH SERVICE:
ENGLAND

Since the Department of Health and Social Security (DHSS) published its document on *The NHS Planning System* in 1976,[1] English-style health planning has become equated with the formal process of preparing strategic (ten-year) and operational (three-year) plans. Indeed, the recent institutionalization of this process is significant and will be described; but the more important health planning efforts in England actually emerged prior to and along with the present NHS planning system.

Immediately following the creation of the NHS in 1948, policymakers attempted to cope with the consequences resulting from nationalization of hospitals and the removal of financial barriers to health care. Having established a system where priorities were to be set on the basis of "medical need" rather than ability to pay, planners had to make major adjustments. By the end of 1948, GPs reported an increase in the demand for their services and more patients were referred to consultants in hospital outpatient departments. In the 1950s, however, successive governments gave priority to housing and education rather than to the NHS.[2] Consequently, there were pressures to control expenditures.

During the early years of the NHS policymakers were responsible not merely for presiding over changes in the administrative organization of health services in accordance with the NHS Act but were also to do this in the face of powerful vested interests and within stringent financial constraints. In this context, NHS planners concentrated their efforts on defending the new arrangements for health care delivery and on avoiding disasters. In the late fifties, as Britain's economy recovered from the war, successive governments allocated an increased portion of annual economic growth to the NHS. In these more prosperous times, NHS planners grew more ambitious. They sought to increase the level and distribution of services. During the seventies, however, the context for health planning changed once again. Largely as a response to increasing health care costs and fiscal crisis, the emphasis of English health policy shifted from simply making services available to providing them in the most effective and efficient way. The result was to strengthen formal planning procedures within the DHSS, first by reorganizing the administrative structure of the NHS and most recently by devising new criteria for resource allocation within the NHS.

ORIGINS AND EARLY YEARS OF HEALTH PLANNING

Before the creation of the NHS, Aneurin Bevan had criticized the lack of planning: "Our hospital organization has grown up with no plan, with no system; it is unevenly distributed over the country and indeed it is one of the tragedies of the situation that very often the best hospital facilities are available where they are least needed."[8]

Following the creation of the NHS, the Ministry of Health (later changed to the DHSS) controlled all but a small proportion of health expenditures. It also appointed members to the regional hospital boards and executive councils, supervised the local health authorities, reviewed the capital building program, issued regulations, devised incentives to improve the distribution of GPs, and ultimately could impose central directives on the NHS. In this institutional setting, one would expect that initial health planning efforts in England played an important role in shaping resource allocation decisions within the health sector. This was not so, however.

Until the early seventies, the Ministry of Health was reluctant to intervene in regional health affairs. Harry Eckstein evaluated the performance of the NHS at the end of its first decade and was struck by the unsystematic quality of its policymaking process. He argued that early NHS planners functioned under conditions that were hardly conducive to "rational planning."[4] Ten years later, George Maddox assessed English policies with respect to the supply of physicians, hospital beds, and health centers and characterized English health planning as a process of "muddling through."[5] It appears that planning objectives were inconsistent, the psychological pressures of working out immediate problems were intense, and despite the new structures of the NHS, as always, planners operated under severe constraints.

The formative years of the NHS were dominated by the problems of integrating former voluntary and municipal hospitals under the newly formed regional hospital boards and by the concern about rising costs. In 1945, Aneurin Bevan had argued that given a well-financed national health service, the population would soon get healthier, the need for services would consequently decrease, and the costs would then go down. The 1946 National Health Service Act estimated the expenditure for England and Wales at £110 million. After the first nine months of the service, however, the annual cost was estimated at £242 million, and this rose to £305 million at the end of 1948. In 1950 the chancellor of the exchequer imposed a ceiling of £352 million for the NHS.[6] Under such financial constraints, long-term planning for hospitals was crippled from the start. Although regional hospital boards had the responsibility for producing plans, the lack of money as well as data made it difficult to take this task seriously. The early NHS planners were, in effect, short-run problem solvers whose time was mostly taken up by budgeting duties and crisis management. As Rudolf Klein put it, "Planning was conspicuous by its absence."[7]

The NHS inherited an obsolete hospital infrastructure. About 45 percent of the beds were in buildings erected before 1891, and 21 percent were in buildings erected before 1861.[8] During the first seven years of the NHS not a single new hospital was built.[9] In the early years of the NHS, capital expenditure in real pounds was equal to about a third of the level of 1938–1939.[10] It was not until 1955 that the government made modest increases in capital expenditures for hospital plant replacement and modernization. At that time, while the level of hospital building expenditure was £10 million, minister of health Iain Macleod extracted a promise of £23 million from the treasury; but that was soon cut back again because of new economic conditions. Until the early sixties, periodic budget allocations for hospital building and modernization were subjected to repeated cutting.

In the 1960s, French-style economic planning spread across the Channel, and the treasury was drawn to the idea of developing long-term strategies as a way of managing the new prosperity. A period of growth began—both in hospital construction and modernization as well as in hospital planning. In 1962, while Enoch Powell was minister of health, a Ten Year Plan for balanced hospital development was produced.[11] This document laid the basis for planning the entire hospital network within the NHS. Its aim was to replace every hospital built before World War II. Furthermore, it advocated the replacement of small rural hospitals with modern district general hospitals, the development of short-stay psychiatric departments within the general hospitals, and the phasing out of large, long-stay psychiatric institutions.

When submitting the Ten Year Plan to Parliament, Enoch Powell remarked at a news conference that "the introduction of the Plan marked one of the most important days of the health service, because it gave the opportunity to plan the hospital service on a scale not possible anywhere else certainly on this side of the 'Iron Curtain.' "[12] The plan called for 90 new hospitals with an average of 600 beds each. In addition, it recommended the remodeling of 134 hospitals as well as 356 major special modernization schemes. All this was estimated to cost £500 million over ten years. In fact it would have cost much more; consequently a more modest version of the plan was actually implemented.

By 1974 only a quarter of district general hospital beds were provided in new or remodeled hospitals, and in 1978, fully one-third of the hospitals had been erected before 1900.[13] Nevertheless, the Ten Year Plan was a significant achievement not only for improving the hospital stock but also for revitalizing one of the central goals of the NHS— rationalization of the health sector. Much like the creation of the NHS, the Ten Year Plan was preceded by a series of government reports that analyzed the key problems in the health sector and proposed comprehensive strategies for change. Indeed, the process of preparing the plan raised fundamental questions about the role of the hospital: How many hospitals should be built per thousand population? How large should they be? And perhaps most important, what is the appropriate balance of services within a community between inpatient and ambulatory care? Although the plan explicitly recognized the important interdependence between local authority services and hospital care and even urged an increase in home care provided by social workers, most of the budgetary allocations for implementing the plan went directly to buildings and thereby encouraged the development of health services away from the GP and the community and toward the hospital.

In addition to planning for hospitals, NHS planners attempted to improve access to and quality of ambulatory care by designing incentives to reduce geographic disparities in the distribution of GPs and by upgrading community services.

Section 34 of the National Health Service Act required the minister to appoint a Medical Practices Committee (MPC) with powers of negative control over the residential settlement of GPs. Since the creation of the NHS, the MPC classified geographic areas according to the average GP list size of enrolled patients in the region. A system of negative direction denied the executive councils the right to accept applications from GPs in "overdoctored" areas (average list size under 1800). This policy was moderately successful as long as the supply of new doctors increased. For example, between 1952 and 1961, the proportion of the population in "underdoctored" areas decreased from 52 to 17 percent. Between 1963 and 1967, however, as the number of GPs declined, the proportion of the population living in underdoctored areas increased again to 38 percent.[14] In 1966, NHS planners introduced a system of positive incentives. Special practice allowances were introduced to encourage physicians to locate in "designated areas" (average list size over 2,500). But Michael Cooper concludes, "In practice, this scheme has had little effect. First the size of the supplement is likely to be only about ten percent of the doctor's expected income and second, doctors tend to work where they do for largely nonmonetary reasons."[15]

From the point of view of planning to upgrade community services—in particular, the construction of health centers—the policy of providing positive incentives had salutary and perhaps even unintended effects. One of the goals of the NHS Act was to promote the organization of general practice in health centers as a way to encourage comprehensive care by linking primary medical services to nursing and community social services. The unwillingness of physicians to work in such centers, combined with the financial stringency of local authorities, however, ensured that few were built in the early years. In 1966, in addition to positive incentives for setting up practice in underdoctored areas, and as part of an agreement between the government and the medical profession (the so-called Charter for the

Family Doctor Service), a flat-rate practice allowance was introduced for any GP with a list size exceeding 1,000 patients. In addition, the General Practice Finance Corporation was established to reimburse the rent for health centers and to make loans to GPs for buying, building, or improving premises. The result was that whereas there were only 30 health centers in all of England and Wales at the end of 1965, by the end of 1973, 523 health centers were open.[16] Unfortunately, health centers have done little more than house GPs either in solo or group practice; or in Brian Abel-Smith's optimistic assessment, by 1973, "one doctor in seven worked in a health center designed to accommodate the basic primary care team, including district nurses and health visitors."[17]

As a plan to increase access by improving the spatial distribution of GPs, the policy of negative and positive incentives in designated areas appears to have been not merely ineffective but ill conceived.[18] Surely the definition of a medically deprived area should transcend merely the statistic of list size. Moreover, the money involved in attracting more physicians to underdoctored areas might be more efficiently spent in hiring ancillary staff, improving practice facilities, or expanding local authority social services. Above all, policy on physician location was and remains uncoordinated among those groups responsible for making influential decisions. The incentives to physicians in underdoctored areas result from negotiations between the British Medical Association (BMA) and the DHSS; the value of the incentives is set by the Review Body on Doctors' and Dentists' Remuneration and is subject to final approval by the government; and the designation of areas to which these incentives apply is determined by the Medical Practices Committee, which has traditionally emphasized its independence of both the BMA as well as the DHSS.

As in France, despite the problems of planning, improvements in the access and quality of ambulatory care, health planning as hospital construction and modernization produced more tangible results. By 1973, NHS planners had built 79 new hospitals and significantly rebuilt or modernized 112 others. In 1974–1975, funds were allocated for 85 major hospital schemes; and in 1975–1976, 33 more were in progress.[19] Between 1953 and 1972, real expenditures on the NHS had increased 130 percent—faster than total public expenditures (83 percent) and slower than education (240 percent) and social security (160 percent). But most of the increase went to the hospital system and preserved existing disparities among levels of hospital provision.[20] As Klein points out, budget allocations during the first fifteen years of the NHS were distributed on the principle of "to him who hath shall more be given: the yearly increments in regional revenue allocations were based largely on existing regional commitments, with the inevitable result of perpetuating inherited inequalities."[21]

The early years of English health planning were based on the assumption that the need for health care was finite. Cooper argues, however, that such an assumption was unfounded:

> Doctors, nurses and other professional groups have increasingly found themselves in the front line of a system which could not deliver what it had seemingly promised. Having set out to provide the impossible, namely the elimination of unmet need, the professions have increasingly found themselves fulfilling the role of assessing relative needs and rationing scarce health resources amongst them.[22]

The ability of hospital consultants to control the allocation of resources at the local level reinforced hospital-centered health care to the detriment of preventive services and caring functions. Moreover, the clinical freedom of physicians to decide on the use of hospital resources limited the power of NHS planners to reallocate health resources away from the hospital to meet the growing number of services required by the elderly and the mentally and chronically ill.

By the late sixties and early seventies, while Britain's

economic crisis created pressures to reduce public expenditures and stimulate private investment, technological developments in medical care combined with England's aging population led to growing claims on the NHS budget. It became increasingly clear to the treasury and to NHS planners that steps would have to be taken to reorganize the NHS in order to make it more responsive to central controls.

HEALTH PLANNING AS REORGANIZATION

In 1974, following the reorganization of local government, the entire structure of the NHS was reorganized, and a formal health planning apparatus was created (fig. 9).[23] The regional hospital boards (RHBs) and nearly all boards of governors (BGs) were abolished and replaced by regional health authorities (RHAs) that became responsible for planning and allocating all health resources within fourteen regions roughly corresponding to the former RHBs.*

These regions were, in turn, subdivided into ninety area health authorities (AHAs) that replaced the former hospital management committees. The AHAs, whose boundaries were aligned with those of the local authorities, are responsible for planning and managing comprehensive health services for an average population of 500,000. To this end, they took over some of the pre-1974 local government services such as ambulances and domiciliary nursing, as well as titular control of the family practitioner committees (FPCs) that replaced the executive councils. Finally, within each AHA, districts were established to serve a population ranging from 80,000 to 500,000. Within this local unit of the new NHS, the district management teams (DMTs) are responsible for identifying health needs, pro-

---

*On April 1, 1982, there was another administrative reorganization of the NHS. This does not, however, alter the basic argument developed in this chapter (see note 65).

The Bevan NHS

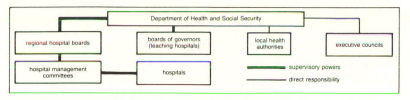

The NHS from 1 April 1974

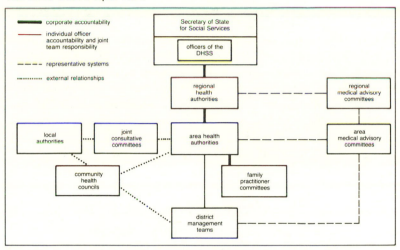

Fig. 9. The administrative reorganization of the NHS.

Source: R. Klein, "A Guide to the New NHS," *New Society* 27, 595 (Feb. 28, 1974), 514–517.

ducing district plans, and day to day management of health services in their district.

This reorganized administrative structure reflects the goals of DHSS policymakers. They sought to unify the NHS by integrating health services both at a local level and at the level of the AHA. In addition, they intended to eliminate the fragmentation of the former tripartite structure and to improve coordination by linking health services provided by the AHA with the social services provided by local authorities. They also wanted to increase local, professional, and consumer participation in the management of the AHA through the joint consultative committees, the professional advisory committees, and the community health councils. Finally, by streamlining management functions and instituting a planning system, DHSS policy-makers sought to increase central control over resource allocation within the NHS.[24]

As R. G. S. Brown points out in his book on *Reorganizing the National Health Service:*

> Planning capacity was regarded as an important feature of the new structure, which would enable rational decisions to be taken about the best use of resources in the face of changing needs, including improvement in the neglected sectors of care and a fairer distribution of resources to different parts of the country. It was hoped that the new structure would itself facilitate planning: the new authorities were responsible for meeting the health needs of their areas across the board, and would be assisted by the new breed of medical administrators. But it was also felt necessary to introduce a new planning process.[25]

The formal process of health planning in the reorganized NHS is well summarized in figure 10 which shows the iterative nature of the task. Strategic (ten-year) considerations as well as operational (three-year) plans are supposed to begin simultaneously at the national and district levels. Two kinds of guidelines orient this process. They may deal with general policies and procedures or they may be more specific by providing indications of resource availability or standards of resource provision. The guidelines dealing with general policies typically focus on priorities among client groups, for example, the mentally ill, the physically handicapped, and the elderly. The guidelines on resource availability typically reflect decisions by the Public Expenditure Survey Committee (PESC)—an interdepartmental committee chaired by the treasury, which sets the level of all department budgets including the DHSS. The budget figures are adjusted for price inflation, and "cash limits" (a maximum threshold for expenditures) have recently been imposed.[26] Once these figures are set,

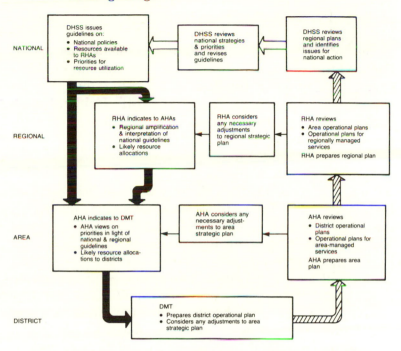

Fig. 10. The flow of guidelines and plans in the NHS.

Source: *The NHS Planning System* (London: DHSS, June 1976), p. 10.

the DHSS, in turn, breaks them down into expenditure allocations for each RHA.

After the guidelines are elaborated by NHS planners, they are formally issued by ministerial circular.[27] The RHAs then adapt them to their own regions and pass down more detailed guidelines to the AHAs and districts. Finally, after a process of negotiation, known as *joint care planning*, between health and local authorities and an elaborate consultation process involving professional advisory committees, community health councils, the AHA, and the district, plans are produced and sent back up the DHSS hierarchy via the RHAs for approval.

The first national experience with this planning cycle took place in the summer of 1976 following the publication of the DHSS document, *The NHS Planning System*. Strategic and operational plans were produced, but they did not always adhere to the priorities and guidelines set by the DHSS. Most often, they consisted of a statement of objectives and a proposal for desired projects rather than an explicit recognition of proposed trade-offs. Planners rarely recommended cutbacks and a reallocation of health resources away from the hospital to community-based services.

Perhaps the most significant aspect of the new NHS planning process was the call for joint care planning and financing.[28] Even before the creation of a single ministry— the DHSS—with responsibility for all health and personal social services, English health policymakers had an interest in coordinating health and welfare resources. The reorganization of local government and of the NHS opened up new opportunities for closer liaison and cooperation by aligning the new area health authorities with the local authorities, by putting a statutory obligation on health authorities and local authorities to collaborate, and by devising new administrative machinery for collaboration— the Joint Consultative Committees (JCC). The JCCs are supposed to allocate responsibility and coordinate services in the shady area between health and social needs. For example, if local planners agree to reduce the number of hospital beds for the chronically ill, *joint financing funds* are supposed to provide for the expansion of more community-based and domiciliary care.

It is probably too early to assess the impact of joint planning. The evidence to date, however, suggests that coordination of health and social services has a long way to go. For example, an evaluation study conducted in West Yorkshire concludes that

> joint planning in Calderdale is now stuck in a rut. The two sides return to the same issues over and over again only to meet the same obstacles to progress as they encountered before— different priorities, lack of money, different views about the nature of the problems and how best to resolve them, different

ideas about the division of responsibilities. In turn, this leads to frustration and disillusionment on both sides, which places an increasingly greater strain on working relations and the credibility of the system. Joint planning is more likely to expire out of weariness than from antagonism. A major initiative is required to break the deadlock. Joint financing acted as just such an impetus but it is not enough to ensure continuing progress. The size of the program is too small, and the squeeze on local government expenditure has made local authorities wary of spending existing monies, never mind larger allocations.[29]

The reasons for this reported failure are hardly surprising when one considers the political, financial, and organizational barriers to success. On the one hand, health and social services are subject to different kinds of political control and public accountability. The reorganized NHS is administered through management tiers, only some of which are, in theory, under the central control of the DHSS. Control of the social service departments, on the other hand, is vested in elected representatives of the local authority. From a financial perspective, health services are centrally controlled, whereas the social service budget— with the exception of certain statutory services—is set by the local authority, which has to meet at least a proportion of this expenditure from locally raised taxes. Furthermore, from an organizational perspective, the health and local authorities operate with different professional perspectives and administrative procedures.

If one were to interpret literally the flow of guidelines and plans in the NHS (see fig. 10), one might be persuaded that the planning process actually results in coherent national policy meticulously spelled out in a series of concrete plans. In a thorough description of the NHS planning system, two English civil servants go one step farther and suggest that "the planning process provides the main means by which the requirements of the law are made explicit and can be monitored in accordance with the Law."[30] Both the simplified figure and this statement, however, mask the kinds of difficulties mentioned above.

Three problems in particular have hindered the NHS planning process.

First, national policies tend to be very general. They are usually not of immediate relevance to local districts that provide the services and that always vary when compared either with the national average or with levels of service elsewhere. Moreover, policies and guidelines concerning the allocation of financial resources have been developed separately from policies for particular client groups.

Second, the structure of the DHSS preserves the separation between the administration of health services and that of social services and social security. In fact, the DHSS document, *The NHS Planning System*, says nothing about the relationship between planning in the NHS and planning in the DHSS as a whole. There are six main administrative groups within the DHSS, all of which engage in some planning (see fig. 11). The subdivisions within these groups, their complex interactions, and the frequent changes to which they succumb, make it difficult to generalize about their contribution to NHS planning; but it seems clear that the planning process is far from rational. Doreen Irving sums up this second problem of planning:

> Although it might be argued that the main concern in developing national priorities is the distribution between client groups and that the distribution between geographical areas is an entirely separate issue, it is clear from the practical experience in the NHS that the two approaches need to be reconciled. The failure of the DHSS to adopt an integrated approach to planning and resource allocation reflects the structure and working of the Department. The Services Development Group works separately from the Regional Group. Service Development and Finance are tenuously linked by PESC [Public Expenditure Survey Committee] and programme budgets, but these are uncoordinated with . . . the work of the Regional Group.[31]

In his description of planning expenditure in England, William Glaser makes a similar observation:

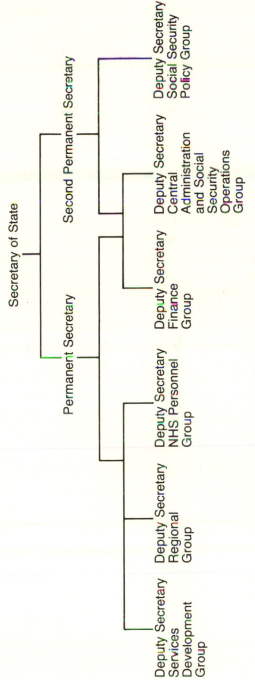

Fig. 11. The permanent and deputy secretaries of the DHSS administrative hierarchy.

Source: M. Butts, D. Irving, and C. Whitt, *From Principles to Practice: A Commentary on Health Service Planning and Resource Allocation in England from 1970 to 1980* (London: Nuffield Provincial Hospitals Trust, 1981), p. 27.

The plans do not match precisely the information fed into the
Finance Division of DHSS when it prepares the Department's
bids for PESC. The strategic and operational plans are written
for entire regions, areas, and districts and not for individual
clinical services. They are designed to treat all medical services
as an integrated complex, pursuant to the philosophy of the
reorganization of 1974. But DHSS itself is organized into
many policy sections, each devoted to one or a few specific
clinical categories such as child health, alcoholism, nutrition,
primary medical care, toxicology, physically handicapped,
dermatology, etc.[32]

The third difficulty that hinders the planning process in
the reorganized NHS is the complex system of formal
consultation on all plans. Districts consult with Community
Health Councils (CHCs), local authorities (LAs), and
district medical committees. And the areas consult with
CHCs, LAs, family practitioner committees, and professional advisory committees. Such participatory processes
are hard to reconcile with the emphasis on central planning
and control.

Above all, and this is the principal argument in this
chapter, the most vulnerable aspect of English health
planning is the gap between the process of setting
guidelines and plans at the national and local levels and the
actual expenditure allocations to achieve implementation at
the local level. As noted in a report to the Royal Commission
on the NHS:

> The control systems consist primarily of financial budgets and
> accounts, and of various controls (e.g., over staffing,
> management costs, and capital works) operated by Health
> Authorities and Health Departments. The financial control
> systems are little used for planning and decision-making in any
> positive sense of resource reallocation or conscious testing of
> alternatives.[33]

Indeed, the reorganization of the NHS succeeded in
creating a structure within which health planning issues are

now widely debated, but it failed to link the process of drawing up local and regional plans to the central determination of priorities and criteria by which to allocate health resources.

HEALTH PLANNING AS RESOURCE ALLOCATION

Two years after the reorganization, national guidelines for resource allocation within the health and social welfare sectors were elaborated. Policy on the development of services for priority groups was outlined in a DHSS consultative document entitled *Priorities for Health and Personal Social Services in England* (the Priorities Document).[34] Policy on the distribution of finance for each RHA was outlined by the Resource Allocation Working Party (RAWP) in a document entitled *Sharing Resources for Health in England* (the RAWP Report).[35] Analysis of both documents reveals a striking lack of coordination between these policies. What is more, the policies sometimes appear to be working at cross-purposes. But most troubling of all, neither document addresses the problem of how the process of national planning could be linked to the actual structure for making decisions.

POLICY ON SERVICE DEVELOPMENT

In March 1975 the regional group within the DHSS issued a letter to regional and area health authorities outlining planning tasks for 1975–1976 and advising them that the Priorities Document would be issued to provide guidelines for service development among client groups. Uncertainty about the level of public expenditures delayed publication of the document until March, at which time the bad news was announced. The Priorities Document began by stating the economic limitations outlined in the White Paper on Expenditure up to 1979–1980. "The level of resources which will be available over the next few years means that difficult choices will have to be made."[36] It went on to explain that capital expenditure would have to be cut back in order to finance expenditures in priority areas: primary care, services for the elderly and physically handicapped, and services for the mentally handicapped and mentally ill. As Barbara Castle, the secretary of state for social services, put it, this strategy involved putting "people before buildings."

The Priorities Document represents the first attempt to devise a national planning strategy both for the DHSS and for social services. Based on a program budget analysis of the NHS, it proposed a projected budget in real terms for 1979–1980 and calculated average rates of increase for major service groupings, which would be necessary to fulfill the recommended priorities (fig. 12). The Priorities Document not only recommended increasing the share of primary-care services from 16.8 to 18.4 percent of total expenditures on health and social services; it explicitly recognized the trade-offs implicit in such a change and therefore recommended decreasing the share of acute and maternity services from 43.1 to 40.7 percent of total NHS expenditures. In addition, the Priorities Document stressed the need to increase the efficiency of existing resources and emphasized community care and services for the elderly, mentally ill, and handicapped rather than hospital care. Moreover, it elaborated the system of service standards first used in the 1962 Hospital Plan and designated new norms of provision, for example, with respect to meeting the needs of the elderly.

In September of 1977 a new DHSS report, *The Way Forward*, continued the debate on priorities. In essence, the new secretary of state for social services, David Ennals, provided further rhetorical support for the principles laid out in the Priorities Document. He drew attention to the importance of NHS planning, joint planning, and what were termed "practical constraints." *The Way Forward* began on an eloquent and crucial note: "The setting of priorities is

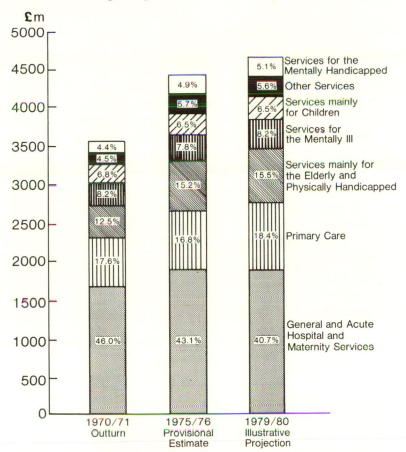

Fig. 12. Expenditure by program as a percentage of total
expenditure current & capital expenditure
(November 1974 prices).

Source: *Priorities for Health and Personal Social Services in England: A Consultative Document* (London: HMSO, 1976), p. 6.

not new; the challenge is to implement them."[37] But beyond
that, it did not address the problem of reconciling strategies
designed to allocate health resources among client groups
and those designed to allocate funds among geographic
regions.

Although both the Priorities Document and *The Way Forward* successfully met their foremost objectives—to state explicitly how health resources might be reallocated and to provoke a debate—they neither indicated how the priorities were to be implemented at the local and regional levels nor provided an ongoing system by which to monitor the pattern of NHS expenditure by client groups. As Peter Fox observed, it is difficult for the central government to know the extent to which regions are following the proposed national priorities since financial management—both in the DHSS as well as within local authorities—is not based on principles of program budgeting.[38] According to the Working Group on Inequalities in Health under the chairmanship of Sir Douglas Black, the Priorities Document actually marks the halt of previous growth in personal and social services. Whereas in 1972–1973 and 1973–1974 expenditures on social services, at constant prices, grew by 15 percent a year, in 1974–1975 and 1975–1976 the rate slowed to 8.3 percent and 6.5 percent, respectively, and became negative in both 1976–1977 and 1977–1978: minus 1.3 and minus 1.6, respectively.[39]

The problem of exercising control over priorities at the local level lies at the root of a central dilemma in English health planning:

> If the central planners insist that their guideline figures should be taken as targets, then they risk imposing a national blueprint even in circumstances where it may be inappropriate or where it may simply be incapable of achievement given local constraints. If, on the other hand, they treat their guidelines simply as a general but not binding indication of what is desirable, then there is a danger that national planning may simply become a rhetorical exercise in persuasion.[40]

At the present time, it appears that English health planning is largely exhortation. Just as the Priorities Document failed to propose an implementation strategy, the RAWP Report failed to link the debate over priorities to resource allocation.

POLICY ON THE DISTRIBUTION OF FINANCE

In March 1975, the DHSS established the Resource Allocation Working Party (RAWP) with a mandate to review arrangements for distributing the financial resources of the NHS to RHAs, AHAs, and districts. The RAWP Report is the most recent response by NHS planners to the problem of geographic disparities in the provision of hospital services in England. To date, it is the most sophisticated attempt in England—and perhaps throughout the world—to devise criteria by which to allocate health resources to assure that there will "eventually be equal opportunity of access to health care for people at equal risk."[41] It also represents a continuing shift away from the use of standards as resource allocators to the use of an areawide rationing system to distribute the financial resources of the NHS.

As early as 1970, the DHSS had introduced an areawide rationing formula to make the distribution of NHS funds to regional authorities more equitable. This "hospital revenue allocation formula" allocated 50 percent of financial resources in proportion to a region's population, 25 percent in proportion to its number of hospital beds, and 25 percent in proportion to its hospital patient treatments (case flows).[42] Since the last two factors reflect the already existing distribution of resources, however, this formula hardly promoted an active redistribution policy, for resource-rich regions automatically received roughly half of the new funds distributed (depending on relative costs) on the basis of already acquired capital. Further, the formula was limited in two other ways. First, it did not tackle the problem of disparities in hospital provision within regions, which are far greater than those between regions.[43] Second, it failed to take account of regional differences in the provision of GP and local authority health services.

The RAWP Report marked a significant advance over former redistribution policy. It proposed a formula to calculate equitable budget allocations—both operating expenditures and capital—to each of the RHAs as well as within RHAs (at the subregional level). To calculate "revenue targets" for each region,[44] health services were classified on the basis of available data into seven service categories: (1) nonpsychiatric inpatient, (2) day-patient and outpatient, (3) community health, (4) ambulance, (5) family practitioner committee (FPC) administration, (6) mental illness inpatient, and (7) mental handicap inpatient. For each category, midyear population estimates were combined in proportion to their relative shares (based on recent national expenditure). Then each service category was weighted by appropriate combinations of factors such as age, sex, marital status, fertility, and standardized mortality ratio (an indicator that reflects the difference between mortality rates in a given RHA and those that apply to the entire population of England). Finally, adjustments were made for cross-boundary flows of patients (i.e., patients who leave their region to receive medical care), service increments for teaching (SIFT) to cover certain additional costs in teaching hospitals, and a number of other factors (fig. 13). At the end of this process, within the total NHS budget available, derived revenue targets for each region were compared to current RHA revenue allocations.

RAWP also provided a method to allocate capital targets, but this is not the place to delve into the accounting details of capital stock valuation. The point is that as in the calculation of revenue targets, the capital allocation formula is also based on the use of weighted populations (with the population base projected five years). And as in the calculation of revenue targets, capital targets were compared to the present regional capital stock to determine the levels of excess or deficit in the share of capital. The RAWP Report proposed that over the decade up to 1986–1987, amounts varying between 10 percent and 30 percent of the total capital budget should be allocated among the regions with a historic capital stock deficit.

With respect to revenue and capital targets, the policy implications were clear. At the time of the RAWP Report in

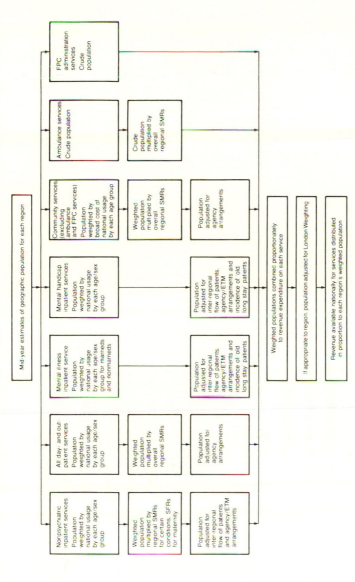

Fig. 13. The components of the revenue* target.

*In English parlance, *revenue* refers to *operating expenditures*.

Source: Department of Health and Social Security, *Sharing Resources for Health in England: Report of the Resource Allocation Working Party* (HMSO, 1976), p. 26.

1976, the analysis indicated that the allocation of NHS funds to the four regions of London (N.E., N.W., S.E., and S.W. Thames) and to Oxford should be decreased by a factor ranging from 1.9 to 14.7 percent while the other nine provincial regions in England should receive increased allocations by a factor ranging from 2.8 to 14.2 percent (fig. 14).[45]

Needless to say, the RAWP solution has attracted considerable attention and generated much controversy. Like all administrative formulas for allocating resources, the RAWP formula raises a number of methodological and conceptual problems.[46]

With respect to method, technical criticisms have been leveled against the use of standardized mortality ratios (SMRs) in the weighting of regional population estimates. More specifically, the assumed linear relationship between SMRs and need has been challenged,[47] but a strong case has also been made for their continued use and the limited budgetary effects of proposed adjustments.[48] In addition,

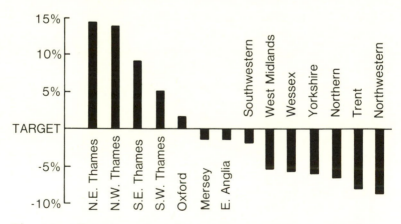

Fig. 14. Allocations to regions as a percentage above or below RAWP targets (RAWP 1976).

Source: Adapted from *Cuts in the NHS* (London: Politics of Health Group, 9 Poland St. London W1), p. 13. The data are from the RAWP Report, *Sharing Resources for Health in England* (London: HMSO, 1976), p. 74.

the problem of cross-boundary flows has provoked debate. A case has been made that more complex and therefore more costly cases will cross boundaries.[49] Further, anomalies arising from the use of *net* cross-boundary flows have been pointed out.[50] Each region, area, and district has its own admission rate and relative hospital costs. But the cross-boundary flow is translated into population equivalents using the national admission rate and, at least until 1978, there were no specialty cost estimates to adjust for variation in hospital costs.

With respect to conceptual problems there are four critical issues. First, the calculation of SIFT allocations provoked vigorous criticism, particularly from London. Time and again, the need to maintain national and international specialty hospitals—"centers of excellence," as they were called—was emphasized. SIFT only provides a special allocation for educational costs. This means that the RAWP Report tended to neglect London's extra costs for medical research and the development of new techniques, the demonstration of higher standards of medical care, and the treatment of complex cases from outside its catchment area.

Second, the FPC component of the RAWP formula's population weightings apply only to administration costs. GP services themselves are funded outside the RAWP formula because of their independent contractor status. This results in a classic case of suboptimization, for GP services are not independent of the burden placed on hospital and community services. The balance between these services is a critical consideration in health planning; and as Buxton and Klein note, if the logic of RAWP were to include the funding of GP services, it would have significant implications for their redistribution.[51]

Third, the RAWP formula weights regional population figures on the basis of recent national utilization among the seven service categories rather than on the basis of the Priorities Document's recommended usage for each category. In this sense the RAWP Report appears to be working at cross-purposes with the Priorities Document.[52] Had the

RAWP formula integrated the Priorities Document planning criteria, its calculation of regional expenditure targets would have been altered.[53] Although the resulting change in allocation would be marginal and although this conceptual defect is admittedly a technical point, it nevertheless indicates a revealing lack of coordination between the formulation of planning criteria for service development among client groups and the RAWP formula's criteria of territorial equity in the distribution of finance.

Fourth, and perhaps most important, are the assumptions made by the RAWP Report. Upon reflection, the notion is really quite fanciful that distributing financial resources to reduce inequality of inputs will actually result in the closing of gaps between output measures such as SMRs.[54] The RAWP solution assumes that equity in the distribution of finance is proportional to equity in the distribution of health resources, which is, in turn, proportional to equity of health service provision. The level of health care provision, however, reflects not merely the quantity of health resources but also depends on what mix of services are deployed, where they are located, and how efficiently they are used. Although the RAWP Report provided a rationale for allocating operating expenditures and capital among geographic regions, it did not—and quite intentionally so—confront the question of how, once health resources are allocated, they ought to be deployed.[55]

In spite of these methodological and conceptual problems, the RAWP Report has exercised a powerful influence on health planning in the NHS. Depending on the growth of the total NHS budget and on the political will to effect change, one of two principal strategies could be adopted to achieve equitable resource allocation in the health sector: (1) a Robin Hood strategy of taking from the rich regions and giving to the poor,[56] or (2) a strategy of differential expansion whereby only increases in the NHS budget are redistributed.

Although the increase in the NHS budget has been barely sufficient to keep up with the additional demands resulting from the aging of the population and the growing sophistication of diagnostic and treatment procedures, the DHSS has rejected the Robin Hood approach in favor of a policy of differential expansion. Clearly, the DHSS has been cautious largely in order to minimize opposition and dislocation of services in the most well-endowed regions. But as indicated in table 10, the implementation of the RAWP Report's proposals has had an impact on regions' revenue allocations since 1976–1977.[57] Over the six years that the RAWP formula has been used as a basis for determining revenue allocations to regions, the London regions and Oxford have received small positive growth rates— most recently as low as .6 percent for the S.W. Thames region.[58] In contrast, the largest percentage change in allocation has been experienced by the N.W. Thames region, which grew from 88 percent in 1976–1977 to 94 percent in 1981–1982.

An estimate from the Social Services Committee suggests

TABLE 10
COMPARISON OF ACTUAL ALLOCATION TO REGIONS
IN ENGLAND WITH TARGET ALLOCATIONS*

	% 1976–1977†	% 1978–1979	% 1981–1982
North Western	88	92	94
Trent	90	93	94
Northern	91	93	95
West Midlands	94	94	96
East Anglia	93	95	95
Wessex	94	96	95
South Western	95	96	95
Yorkshire	96	97	96
Mersey	98	98	100
Oxford	107	102	100
S.W. Thames	108	106	106
S.E. Thames	116	112	109
N.E. Thames	116	114	110
N.W. Thames	117	114	115

Source: Finance Division DHSS (London, February 1981).
*Percentages reflect proportion that actual allocation bears to target allocation.
†Financial years end March 31.

that the process of reaching all RAWP targets will take at least ten years.[59] This is not surprising given the slow overall growth of the NHS, the imposition of cash limits, and political pressures, notably from the Thames regions. What is more surprising, however, is the failure to link policy on service development to policy on the distribution of finance.

POLICY INTEGRATION AND IMPLEMENTATION

By providing the criteria that serve to distribute future funding to RHAs, the RAWP Report is a strategic component in the NHS planning process. Indeed, the implementation of areawide and local plans depends on the way in which RAWP calculations are applied. A rational approach to planning the allocation of health resources in England would suggest the integration of policy on service development with policy on the distribution of finance. But as we have seen, these policies are fundamentally different, and the DHSS has made no attempt to reconcile them. The RAWP Report emphasizes territorial equity in the distribution of finance; the Priorities Document and *The Way Forward* emphasize service provision among client groups.

The failure to integrate parallel policies raises serious questions about the state of English health planning. At the level of central government, because the DHSS bases its financial allocations on the RAWP formula, regional health plans are never regarded as representing competing strategies for the use of available NHS resources. As a consequence, within regions, policies on service development that are inconsistent with DHSS guidelines can be pursued without jeopardizing financial allocations. The same applies at the subregional level, where linking service development policy with finance is crucial to achieve implementation of planning goals. For example, in the N.E. Thames region the distribution of funding did not prevent local planners from cutting acute hospital services mainly through a reduction in the number of long-term stay beds serving largely the poor and the elderly.[60]

An analysis by Tom Rathwell in 1981 revealed that the priorities and guidelines set by the DHSS are not, in practice, being endorsed by the regions.[61] Contrary to what NHS planners wish, financial incentives at the local level do not reinforce and often go against the implementation of national objectives. For example, despite joint planning activities and NHS efforts at "pump priming" through joint financing of certain social services, there is little planners can do to incite AHAs and local authorities to revise their current expenditure patterns. Further, since most of the budget for primary care provided by GPs is met directly by the DHSS, it is impossible locally to transfer resources from family practitioner committees (FPCs) to AHAs or districts and vice versa. Consequently, AHAs or districts that are short of GPs cannot get money to spend on substitutable services, and AHAs have neither management responsibilities nor incentives to control FPC spending, thereby altering the configuration of health services. Needless to say, this is a structural weakness of the NHS, and even the most successful efforts at policy integration would not be sufficient to correct it.

EVALUATION OF ENGLISH HEALTH PLANNING

Health planning as reorganization succeeded in creating a new administrative structure and in institutionalizing a formal planning process. Health planning as resource allocation succeeded in making the central government explicitly recognize trade-offs among alternative resource configurations within the health sector. Neither kind of planning, however, has succeeded in achieving policy integration and implementation. Regional disparities in the provision of health care services remain, whether measured in terms of expenditures, hospital beds, or manpower. The priorities outlined in the Priorities Document and in *The Way Forward* remain unmet. And the NHS remains a health service characterized by hospital-centered care.[62]

Despite the 1974 reorganization, NHS planners have so

far failed to unify the tripartite structure and to influence, in the best interest of the population, the distribution of the NHS budget among categories of health care. Although the geographical boundaries between AHAs and local authorities were aligned, the jurisdictional responsibilities still overlap with regard to the provision of certain social services, particularly to the elderly and the mentally ill. Although FPCs were made accountable to AHAs, they still remain what Klein calls an "autonomous enclave within the NHS," for GPs have maintained their status as independent contractors. The ironic result is that NHS planners have the least amount of administrative control over precisely those sectors which they wish to influence most: social services and primary medical care.

Although the reorganization succeeded in increasing central and managerial control over the NHS, it also strengthened professional consultative machinery and created a number of representative institutions for increasing the role of consumers and NHS workers in making local decisions. The result has often been a situation of stalemate, in which either participatory mechanisms weed out controversial issues from the agenda or central guidelines are resisted, delayed, and even blocked. Why, for example, should AHAs accept centrally determined priorities if they involve service cutbacks and loss of jobs? How can AHAs expect to implement their own health plans when physicians have "clinical freedom" to make decisions that commit most of an AHA's resources?

Such questions reflect some of the key problems of health planning in the NHS. The most crucial problem, however, is the failure to achieve policy integration and implementation by linking central planning guidelines directly to the financing of health and social services. As the RAWP formula is refined, it is likely to be relied on more closely than it was over the last six years as the most equitable basis by which to distribute scarce financial resources. As the role of RAWP in resource allocation increases, given the present trend in the NHS toward administrative devolution, the

DHSS is also likely to find it increasingly difficult to influence directly priorities at subregional levels. Thus, in order to assure implementation of national priorities and health plans, policy analysts argue that the processes of planning and funding in England must be fused.[63] In 1979 the Royal Commission on the NHS accepted this view: "We agree with the Expenditure Committee that: 'the expenditure planning and priority setting of DHSS should be synchronized so as to enable Parliament to examine the relationship between the two.' "[64] This aspect of English health planning is likely to receive careful scrutiny in the years to come.[65]

PART IV

COMPARATIVE
EVALUATION AND
CONCLUSIONS

8

HEALTH PLANNING: AMERICAN STYLE

In comparison with France, Québec, and England, the United States provides an example of more flexible and decentralized health planning efforts. The problems, however, are no different from those discussed in the case studies. They involve balancing needs and resources and linking health planning to health care financing so that reimbursement incentives induce the implementation of health plans.

Political discourse on health planning in the United States has focused on the conventional opposition between plan and market, regulation and competition. It is increasingly clear, however, that policy goals, such as controlling rising health care costs, are unlikely to be implemented without recourse to both regulation and competition and without more explicit efforts to link health planning to health care financing.

This chapter makes a case for improving health planning practice in the United States. First, it reviews and evaluates the evolution of health planning efforts in the United States. Then it considers alternative strategies for health planning in light of the current debate over encouraging competition and eliminating the formal health planning system.

CENTRAL PROBLEMS AND EARLY HEALTH
PLANNING EFFORTS

Federal interest in health planning issues may be attributed to three central problems: (1) inequitable access to health services, (2) uneven quality of health services, and (3) rapidly mounting health care costs.

First, despite Medicare and Medicaid, studies suggest that access to health services is highly correlated with socio-economic, cultural, and geographic factors.[1] Large disparities persist in the geographic distribution of physicians and hospitals. States unevenly finance a variety of poorly balanced programs. For example, there are large discrepancies in the level of Medicaid payments between California and Mississippi. In addition, health services are fragmented. There are no clear entry and exit points in the health system, and the categorical programs for the poor assure neither continuity of care nor equitable access to services.[2]

Second, the quality of medical care varies among states and even within states. To cite only one example, after adjusting for income, occupation, age, and sex, a study in Vermont revealed wide discrepancies in the utilization of surgical services between small areas.[3] Tonsillectomies ranged from 4 to 41 per 1,000 children per year. Hysterectomies ranged from 30 to 60 per 10,000 women per year. There is additional evidence of such disparities in the provision of care throughout the country. Also, questions have been raised about the impact of medical care on health status. Only in recent years have systematic efforts emerged to evaluate the results of particular medical procedures and to assess the relative importance of medical care as opposed to public health programs in achieving particular health impacts.[4]

Third, as is true for most other nations, costs in the United States have soared. Per capita annual health care costs rose from $426 to $975 between 1965 and 1981.[5] The government share (federal and state) of total health expenditures rose from 20 percent to 40 percent after the passage and implementation of Medicare and Medicaid.[6] Employers, who finance a large portion of private health insurance premiums, have had to pay higher premiums to maintain agreed-upon levels of medical benefits. As a result, business coalitions have developed to lobby for legislative remedies and to negotiate with health care providers and insurers. In this economic context, labor unions now find it more difficult to negotiate real direct wage increases. No wonder that government, employers, and labor unions agree on the need for containing the rate of increase of health care costs.

Early health planning activities in America were largely voluntary efforts to agree on priorities for the allocation of capital funds resulting from community hospital fund drives and local philanthropy. The first major effort of the federal government to promote health planning began with the Hill-Burton Hospital Survey and Construction Act in 1946.[7] To qualify for federal subsidies available for hospital construction and modernization, each state was required to submit a health plan containing detailed resource inventories in the health sector and estimates of need. The funds were provided to the states by the federal government on the basis of a formula, and the states, in turn, provided direct grants to the hospitals.

As in France, Québec, and England, at first, health planning efforts in the United States concentrated on hospital construction and modernization. By the mid-sixties, hospitals in almost all metropolitan areas of the United States were receiving some kind of federal subsidy under the Hill-Burton Act. Moreover, in 1965, the Heart Disease, Cancer, and Stroke Amendments created Regional Medical Programs in fifty-six regions.[8] This legislation aimed at speeding up the application of new biomedical knowledge by providing subsidies for regional cooperative arrangements that emphasized training of medical personnel and improved links between medical schools, teaching hospitals, and community hospitals.

In addition to the Hill-Burton funds, because of the

favorable reimbursement policies of Medicare, Medicaid, and private health insurance, most hospitals were able to secure private loans for their expansion and modernization. By the 1970s these loans paid for through higher per diem rates surpassed the level of direct government subsidies to hospitals. As a result, the number of hospitals grew and many were successfully modernized. But inequitable access, uneven quality, and soaring costs resulted in still other attempts to rationalize the health care system.

American policymakers responded to the central problems outlined above by a series of ad hoc legislative measures, most of which were aimed at containing health sector growth through expanded health planning efforts and government regulation of the health system.

HEALTH PLANNING AS A STRATEGY OF DECENTRALIZED INTERVENTION

The essence of the new approach to health planning and regulatory control may be characterized, with hindsight, as a strategy of decentralized intervention that was largely unrelated to provider reimbursement policies. In summary, this strategy (1) required states and local areas to produce comprehensive health plans, (2) created organizations to review professional standards of hospital care, (3) developed limited regulatory controls over hospitals to avoid unnecessary duplication of facilities, (4) encouraged the organization of prepaid medical care organizations as an alternative to conventional fee-for-service practice, and (5) reorganized and expanded health planning functions by creating new regional, state, and local health planning agencies.

THE COMPREHENSIVE HEALTH PLANNING (CHP) ACT

Passed in 1966, this measure required states and local communities to produce health plans.[9] Under the new legislation, CHP agencies produced systematic inventories of health resources. They compared the results with national averages and local plans, made public issues out of the disparities, and proposed broad system changes. Most health plans indicated that excess capacity existed in the hospital sector.[10] There existed duplication in the provision of expensive medical technology and low occupancy rates in numerous hospitals. In contrast, provision of primary medical care was usually found to be lacking in many areas, and there were poor institutional links between primary care services and secondary and tertiary inpatient hospital services.

In their efforts to be comprehensive, the CHP agencies encouraged broad thinking about the components of a health system. They provoked discussions among health professionals, consumers, and administrators and produced some noteworthy blueprints for health sector reorganization. But health planners had limited data and analytic skills for evaluating the health system and virtually no authority for implementing their plans.

THE PROFESSIONAL STANDARDS REVIEW ORGANIZATION (PSRO)

Legislation passed by Congress in 1972 created PSROs to monitor services provided to Medicare and Medicaid beneficiaries. This legislation was a response largely to the pressures for cost containment but also to the need to evaluate the quality of hospital care.[11] By 1974, 203 local PSROs were established throughout the United States, and incentives were created to enlist at least 25 percent of the physicians in each PSRO region as members of the new organization. The task of these physicians is to assess the "necessity" and the "appropriateness" of hospital care for all Medicare and Medicaid beneficiaries.

PSROs have undertaken this task in a variety of ways. Audits have been established to regulate hospital admissions and lengths of stay for particular diagnostic categories. Detailed studies have also been initiated to devise protocols for review of medical care, to evaluate the impact of medical procedures, and to create a uniform data base with which to compare medical practice among regions. Unfortunately, however, PSROs have had uneven success in reducing unnecessary hospital utilization and in altering the practice patterns of physicians providing poor quality care. Although they have resolved neither the problem of uneven quality nor that of mounting costs, it must be recognized that PSROs have provided opportunities for fruitful health services research. They have produced new data sources and improved our capability to evaluate the quality of medical care—all of which will be fundamental in future health planning efforts.[12]

REGULATORY CONTROLS OVER HOSPITALS

Meanwhile several states introduced legislation to curb unnecessary expansion of facilities. These so-called certificate of need (CON) laws regulated hospital expansion programs and capital expenditures above a specific threshold (typically $150,000). New York adopted the first law in 1964, Rhode Island and Maryland followed in 1968, and Connecticut and California in 1969.

At the federal level, as well, Congress adopted the concept of regulating hospital expansion. Section 1122 of the 1972 Amendments to the Social Security Act stipulates that federal funds under Medicare, Medicaid, or Maternal and Child Health may not be used to support unnecessary capital expenditures.[13] States were encouraged to review capital expenditures of health facilities. All organizations engaging in such expenditures without prior approval of the state's designated 1122 planning agency would receive reduced reimbursement for services provided under Medicaid and Medicare. By 1978 the certificate of need was a precondition to licensure in thirty-eight states.

In addition to CON legislation, by 1977 nine state

governments introduced the equivalent of public utility control over the determination of hospital reimbursement . rates.[14] Rate setting bodies generally include representatives of industry, labor, health care institutions, and third-party payers. Their purpose is to ensure that hospital reimbursement rates reflect resource costs, and that all third-party payers accept regulated rates as the basis for hospital reimbursement.

Although there is a good deal of variation among state rate-setting programs, particularly in the methods used to fulfill their mandates, generally the four functions of all rate-setting programs are: (1) review and approve hospital rates on a prospective basis; (2) require uniform reporting of hospital information; (3) require the disclosure of hospital financial information to the public; and (4) review contracts between third-party payers (government programs, Blue Cross, Blue Shield, and commercial insurers).

THE HEALTH MAINTENANCE ORGANIZATION (HMO) ACT

In 1973 Congress passed the HMO Act, which provides federal subsidies to new HMOs to encourage their growth.[15] In contrast to the predominant fee-for-service system of physician remuneration, HMOs and other prepaid group practice organizations assume a contractual responsibility to provide or ensure the delivery of a range of health services in return for a fixed payment from enrolled members. Depending on the kind of HMO model, physicians work either on a fee-for-service or a salaried basis. Such an incentive structure discourages inappropriate or excessive use of ancillary services and of inpatient facilities while at the same time maintaining incentives for quality: an HMO whose subscribers are disappointed may suffer from disenrollment and find it more difficult to attract new members.

The recent development of HMOs was part of a national strategy to reorganize the supply structure of health services. As a competitive alternative to conventional fee-for-service practice, HMOs were intended to provide a system of prepaid medical care that would lead to significant cost savings. In a comprehensive review of empirical studies on cost savings by HMOs, Harold Luft concludes that total health care costs for members have been 10 to 40 percent below costs for those with conventional insurance. In addition, excluding maternity cases, the annual hospitalization rate per 1,000 members has been reduced in some circumstances to less than half that of subscribers in Blue Cross and Blue Shield plans.[16] It is not clear whether HMOs succeed in controlling costs through more appropriate use of services, through greater use of preventive services, or because they enroll a healthier population than other insurance plans.

Under the HMO Act, nonprofit sponsoring organizations can obtain grants to study the feasibility of establishing HMOs. Further, newly operating nonprofit programs can obtain loans to cover deficits during start-up periods, and profit oriented programs can obtain federal guarantees of loans. A crucial feature of the new law is the requirement that a firm with more than twenty-five workers, which provides health care coverage as a fringe benefit, has to offer its employees a choice between conventional health insurance coverage and membership in an HMO if a federally qualified plan exists in the area. In return, the new HMO is required to offer a broad range of benefits and to allow an annual open enrollment period during which all applicants (including those at high risk) are accepted.[17]

THE 1974 HEALTH PLANNING AND RESOURCES DEVELOPMENT ACT

Despite the various initiatives summarized above, in 1974 the planning act declared that the history of public and private sector responses to the problems of inequitable access and rising costs "have not resulted in a comprehensive rational approach to the present problems."[18]

The planning act tried to correct this situation by creating new institutions—Health Systems Agencies (HSAs)—to reinforce the existing network of formal health planning machinery. From the CHP agencies, HSAs took over the function of making local health plans. Several other changes were made in planning organization, including the establishment of a National Health Planning and Resources Development Council to advise Congress and the executive branch, and the creation of five Regional Centers for Health Planning to provide technical assistance to the planning agencies. State Health Planning and Development Agencies (SHPDAs) as well as State Health Coordinating Councils (SHCCs) were also formed to produce and approve statewide health plans.

At the local levels, a network of HSAs was established. As of January 1981, of the 203 agencies designated by the secretary of the Department of Health and Human Services (DHHS), 180 were private nonprofit institutions and 23 were based in public regional bodies or in local government units. Each HSA is required to have a governing board with 51 to 60 percent of its members consumers as opposed to health care providers. Finally, each HSA must produce two planning documents: a five-year resource development plan to be reviewed and updated at least once every three years and an annual implementation plan. To do this, HSAs are responsible for collecting and analyzing data concerning the health status of the residents of its area and the health resources available to them.

The SHPDA is responsible for coordinating each state's health planning activities and for preparing preliminary documents for the elaboration of a state health plan. It also serves as a link to the DHHS and is responsible for final decisions recommended by CON and Section 1122 reviews. Since 60 percent of SHCC members are appointed by the state governor, it is a public policymaking organization more politically sensitive than the technically oriented SHPDA. That explains, perhaps, why it is responsible for the final preparation of the State Health Plan as well as for reviewing federal entitlement programs that involve health resources in more than one health service area.

EVALUATION OF HEALTH PLANNING
IN THE UNITED STATES

In some respects there has been extraordinary progress during the past twenty years in the development of health services and programs in the United States. Hospitals have been expanded and improved. There are effective insurance plans and prepaid medical programs. More people have access to health services. The system is flexible and decentralized. There are more regulatory procedures to avoid duplication of facilities or expansion beyond reasonable requirements. There have been substantial improvements in information systems and in the planning of programs for the future. Nonetheless, health planners and policymakers face a predicament. They are unable to control costs and resource allocations and they are unable to steer the health system in the direction of health planning goals. To a large extent, this problem stems from the fact that some of the key motivations and incentives that shape the behavior of medical care providers tend to be inconsistent with the goals of health planners. To make matters worse, as in France, Québec, and England, the activities of health planning in the United States are separate from those of health care financing.

At the national level, for example, the Health Care Financing Administration (HCFA) coordinates public financing of health services (Medicare and Medicaid), whereas most national health planning activities are conducted separately within the Health Resources Administration (HRA) and within federal facilities and programs such as Veterans Administration hospitals and the Indian Health Service. Before HCFA assumed the health care financing responsibilities of the Social Security Administration, a former director of the Bureau of Health Planning, Eugene Rubel, noted:

> One of the major problems facing us, at HEW, is the rather wide communications gap that exists between the Social Security Administration and the Public Health Service. . . . The financing arm must learn more about health care delivery and the delivering arm must learn more about health care financing.[19]

The same applies at state and local government levels. HSAs carry out planning activities separately from state-owned and municipal hospitals and from rate-setting agencies and third-party payers that reimburse health care providers. Consequently, as Harvey Sapolsky observed, they are "divorced from the responsibilities of paying for the health services that approved projects generate," all of which has led to a situation of "representation without taxation."[20] Consumers and providers are represented on HSA boards as well as in SHPDAs and on SHCCs but rate-setting agencies and third-party payers are not represented.

In evaluating the planning act, Katherine Bauer observed that it

> excludes from the purview of the agencies it creates most of the key elements that currently determine the way the U.S. health system actually operates. Physicians and other health professionals continue to function just as autonomously as before, the basic way the system is financed continues unchanged, and the new review and regulatory functions prescribed by the Act are simply superimposed on the existing complicated regulatory structure, not integrated with it.[21]

In an attempt to improve the operating efficiency of hospitals, the planning act did authorize continuation of experiments with incentive reimbursement mechanisms for hospitals.[22] Still other measures (e.g., the 1972 Social Security Amendments, the Health Maintenance Act of 1973, and the Carter administration's Hospital Cost-Containment Bill) may be cited as part of a legislative strategy to alter financial incentives in health care reimbursement.[23] But despite these small steps, health planning and regulatory activities in the United States remain separated from the activities of third party payers such as HCFA, Blue

Cross, Blue Shield, and commercial insurers.

There is also a wide range of flaws in the administrative arrangements and the conceptual foundations of the planning act.[24] One set of issues involves representation. Consumer majorities on HSA boards are not always representative of their area population, and even when they reflect the sociodemographic characteristics of the population they are supposed to represent, there are no institutional mechanisms to hold them accountable.[25] In contrast, provider representatives on HSA boards are accountable to their powerful constituencies. As a general rule, physicians and hospitals can mobilize significant political resources while consumers lack organizational clout and leadership.[26]

Another issue concerns the impact of the new health planning machinery. The making of plans has proved both controversial and difficult to implement. There have been persistent differences of opinion in the preparation of plans and over issues of bureaucratic turf. A notable example is the difficulty of forging links with PSROs and rate-setting agencies.[27] Worse still, the overwhelming evidence in the literature evaluating HSAs, CON, and Section 1122 programs is that these measures have been ineffective in controlling health care costs.[28]

In their documents and project review hearings, health planners in the United States have repeatedly summarized the present consensus on how resources should be reallocated within the health sector. As in France, Québec, and England, they have often challenged the predominant medical model of hospital-centered care and encouraged development of new resources for community-based health and social services, for public health services, and for occupational health programs. Despite the comprehensive scope of the legislation enacted in 1974 and earlier, however, the authority given to HSAs, SHPDAs, and SHCCs has been insufficient to enable them to implement their plans. Moreover, the financial incentives that underlie the health system currently work at cross-purposes with the guidelines elaborated in HSA plans.

The measures adopted—CHP, CON and Section 1122, PSROs, HMOs, and HSAs—were uniquely American in concept and style. Their most distinguishing feature was their federal character and decentralized administration: national guidelines have been elaborated and supervised by several federal agencies including HRA and HCFA, but the administrative machinery is most highly developed at state and local levels. Because health planning in the United States operates within a system characterized by diverse sources of financing and pluralistic organizational structures, there is a potential for social experiments (demonstration projects), organizational innovations such as HMOs, decentralized approaches to health care delivery, and the design of new institutional machinery to assure consumer representation. These very virtues, however, make it exceedingly difficult for health planners, particularly at the national level, to influence the allocation of health resources.

ALTERNATIVE STRATEGIES FOR HEALTH PLANNING: COMPETITION, REGULATION, AND REGULATED COMPETITION

The 1979 Amendments to the National Health Planning and Resources Development Act presaged the current debate in America over the relative virtues of competition and regulation as effective strategies for cost containment.[29] A new health planning mandate was established in Section 1502 of the amended legislation:

> The strengthening of competitive forces in the health services industry wherever competition and consumer choice can constructively serve . . . to advance the purposes of quality assurance, cost effectiveness, and access.[30]

HSAs were assigned a new goal—to preserve and improve competition in the health service area—and a new data function, to collect and disseminate the charges for the twenty-five most frequently used hospital services. As noted by the House Committee on Interstate and Foreign Commerce,

> the market forces affecting institutional health services are sufficiently diminished that planning agencies should play a role in allocating the supply of those services. If, however, an innovative financing, reimbursement or service delivery arrangement affecting institutional health services, were designed so that the method of payment by patients (1) created incentives for patients to respond to prices charged and (2) placed the providers at financial risk for unnecessary or excessive services; the committee would expect that planning agencies would, in awarding certificates of need, consider whether the effect of that new arrangement will be to properly allocate the supply of those services. The committee expects that these types of new arrangements would likely involve a population enrolled with a provider on a prepaid basis for the delivery of a comprehensive range of services, including institutional health services.[31]

Since the 1979 amendments to the planning act, five procompetition bills for reform of the health system were introduced in the Ninety-sixth Congress.[32] In addition, the Reagan administration has embraced what it has called the competition strategy. In promoting its view that national regulatory programs should be dismantled, the administration has argued that the planning act and its regulatory mechanisms—in spite of the 1979 amendments—inhibit market forces needed to strengthen competition and consequently should be eliminated. Both the legislative bills, and the Reagan administration's position have been inspired by the work of Paul Ellwood, Clark Havighurst, Walter McClure, and probably most of all by Alain Enthoven's Consumer Choice Health Plan (CCHP), which was originally proposed to DHHS Secretary Joseph Califano in 1977.[33]

The Competition Strategy

The competition strategy would be a striking departure from the way in which France, Québec, and England organize and pay for health care. In contrast to France's national control over reimbursement mechanisms, Québec's prospective annual budgets for hospitals, and England's national health service, advocates of the competition strategy propose to restructure the health sector through the equilibrating forces of the market mechanism.

The competition strategy can be traced to the conservative perspective on the proper role of the state in society (chap. 2). It assumes that the market is the ideal resource allocator and that state intervention should be kept to a strict minimum. In theory, should the state intervene in the health sector, proponents of the competition strategy favor the use of market incentives as opposed to administrative and moral incentives, for example, regulation and exhortation (see table 6). In practice, of course, they favor a combination of policy instruments so long as their objectives are met.

What objectives do proponents of the competition strategy seek? Above all, cost control. Enthoven, for example, calls his health care plan "the only practical solution to the soaring cost of medical care."[34] To achieve this objective, he does not go as far as recommending the elimination of medical licensure as in the free enterprise model advocated by Milton Friedman. Rather, he proposes a plan to restructure the health sector based on four principles of health care financing: (1) multiple choice provision for consumers, (2) fixed dollar subsidies for consumers, (3) uniform rules for qualified health plan competitors, and (4) organization of physicians into competing economic units.

The first two principles focus on the consumption of health services. Consumers would be offered the choice of enrolling in any of the qualified health plans (conventional insurance plans or HMO-type delivery modes) in the area. They would receive a fixed dollar subsidy (voucher) independent of the plan chosen, and would therefore confront the trade-offs between the terms of enrollment (premiums, flat fees, coinsurance and/or deductibles) and the level and range of service benefits provided.

The second two principles focus on the provision of health services. Providers would be required to organize themselves into "competing economic units" capable of delivering a comprehensive range of health services. In addition, providers would be required to conform to uniform rules governing enrollment and premium-setting practices, minimum benefit packages, catastrophic health insurance protection, information disclosure, quality of care, and so on. They would be free to price their services at any level, but consumers would be required to use their vouchers to prepay a fixed annual fee to the plan of their choice for at least the minimum benefit package.

One of the foremost claims for the competition strategy is its political feasibility. Enthoven says the model already exists and works well in some areas of the United States. For example, the Federal Employees' Health Benefit Program offers an annual choice to employees among a variety of private insurance plans (Blue Cross, Blue Shield, Aetna) and numerous HMOs. Employees receive a fixed-dollar subsidy (equal to 60 percent of the average of the premiums of the six largest plans) toward the plan of their choice. Other examples include the growth of competing HMOs in northern California and in the Twin Cities of Minnesota.

However favorable the impact of competition on health care costs is alleged to be, it may be misleading to draw inferences about the political feasibility of the competition strategy from these experiences alone. The reason is that HMOs in existing pockets of competition are not presently constrained to eliminate preferred risk selection of their enrolled members; nor are they constrained to train specialized medical personnel or to finance biomedical research. Physicians and institutional providers currently organized as "competing economic units" depend on their surrounding health care institutions and government programs to train physicians, finance research, and cover high risk populations. In California, for example, preliminary evidence suggests that "competition" may be leaving Blue Cross and Blue Shield plans with an increasingly aging and high cost segment of the population.[35]

If the competition strategy were seriously pursued on a national scale, Enthoven's *Health Plan* suggests ways of dealing with these issues. For example, with respect to problems of preferred risk selection Enthoven proposes rules governing enrollment practices. As for financing teaching and research costs, Enthoven proposes to resolve this problem "through identification of the incremental costs of teaching and research and through direct public subsidies to support these activities at the level considered appropriate by society as determined in the democratic process."[36]

No nation, as yet, has organized its entire health care delivery system on the principles of the competition strategy. One reason, doubtless, is that market competition is not particularly attractive to those "price-takers" who have to compete. In the United States, in spite of the predominant belief in free enterprise and self-equilibrating markets, the leading industrial sectors have more in common with models of oligopoly than with more conventional textbook models of competing producers such as Italian shoe manufacturing. In the health sector, capital is concentrated, collective bargaining between labor unions and hospitals is well developed, consumer ignorance is enormous, the hospital industry is powerful, and physician monopoly power is well recognized. Thus, there remain arguments in favor of regulatory policies so that the state can balance the power of concentrated interests in the health sector.

THE REGULATION STRATEGY

The regulation strategy can be traced to the liberal perspective on the proper role of the state in society (chap. 2). It assumes that practical state intervention is essential for purposes of redressing market failures. In theory, proponents of the regulation strategy favor the use of administrative incentives as opposed to market and moral incentives (see table 6). In practice, like proponents of the competition strategy they are prepared to accept a combination of policy instruments so long as their objectives are met.

In contrast to the proponents of competition, who mainly seek to achieve cost control, proponents of regulation have historically pursued equity as well. To their critics this aim is not altogether realistic and the methods proposed to achieve it are considered naive. Enthoven compares regulation to "trying to make water run uphill."[37] The goals appear impractical, for they run counter to economic incentives and they presuppose an ability to discipline more powerful interests. The evidence we have examined in the case studies supports some of these views and casts doubt on others.

Within a system of cost-based reimbursement of hospitals, as in France, regulation of hospital-day rates has not been effective in controlling rising health care costs. Within systems of fee-for-service physician reimbursement, as in France and Québec, regulation of fees has not controlled the incentives to increase the number of medical procedures, particularly those of a specialized nature. More generally, since the health system tends to be responsive to concentrated provider interests, it was naive to expect regulation of hospital budgets, as in Québec and England, to reallocate significantly resources between hospitals and community-based ambulatory care. In both Québec and England, however, regulation of hospital investment and capital expenditures has succeeded in containing rising health care costs. And regulation of physician fees under NHI in France as well as in Québec, has significantly improved equity of access to services by eliminating financial barriers to medical care.

As noted in chapter 3, the literature on implementation emphasizes the problems of governmental decision making, the complexities of organizational politics, and the general difficulties of "getting things done." Such analyses most often conclude by recommending that government do less—for example, deregulate. An alternative approach, however, is to examine the uses of what Stuart Altman and Sanford Weiner call "regulation as a second best" strategy:

> Conventional planning and regulatory strategies often fail because they focus on constraining only the outputs of the medical system. They tend to assume simple motivations for the regulators and ready compliance by those regulated— ignoring the powerful and contrary incentives an open-ended reimbursement system may offer to both groups. In contrast, we believe that the effectiveness of regulation can be greatly enhanced by a strategy explicitly designed to change those incentives which influence hospitals, physicians and local regulators.[38]

In summary, to make the regulation strategy effective, it is necessary first to adjust the financial incentives that currently drive the health system toward costly hospital-based, technology-intensive medicine and away from community-based primary care services as well as from prevention, occupational, and social service programs.

REGULATED COMPETITION

Much spirited rhetoric has turned the competition-regulation debate into a choice between polar opposites. The competition-regulation dichotomy is quite misleading, however. Enthoven concedes this point by calling his apologia for competition *Health Plan*! His competition strategy, after all, will not come about by the countless decisions of the "Invisible Hand" but by careful evaluation of how to restructure health care organization and financing, that is, planning efforts that then must be firmly embedded into federal regulations and enforced vigorously.

The alternative to regulation is not unalloyed competition, for this ideal is badly thwarted in mainstream American medicine. In rural areas, patients have little choice of hospitals or physicians. In cities, most patients are restricted to the institutions where their physicians prefer to work and have staff privileges. There is virtually no information available to consumers about the relative success of physicians in handling particular patient ailments. Consumers are also not equipped to make decisions based on price and quality. Licensure of medical professionals severely restricts entry into the professions and controls the delegation of tasks among paraprofessionals. Finally, the key decisions that engender health care costs—choice of hospitalization, surgical and diagnostic procedures, and length of hospital stay—remain in the physician's hands.

In effect, the politically feasible alternative to the regulation strategy is not the competition strategy but a strategy that would more properly be termed "regulated competition."

In response to potential perversities in the competition strategy—problems of preferred risk selection, inadequate benefit packages, and marketing abuses by "fly-by-night" HMOs—Enthoven proposes designing "rules" to govern enrollment and premium-setting practices, minimum benefit packages, quality of health care and, more generally, methods of uniform information disclosure by all competing economic units. Unfortunately, however, Enthoven elaborates on neither the proposed rules and regulations nor the mechanisms to determine them, let alone enforce them.

The Omnibus Budget Reconciliation Act of 1981 represents an important step in allowing states the possibility of developing their own rules and regulations to promote competition in the health sector, particularly with regard to the administration of medicaid programs. For example, states now have greater authority to determine eligibility and benefits, to move away from cost-based hospital reimbursement, and to negotiate competitive contracts for some services. In addition, this legislation authorized the secretary of health and human services to waive a variety of statutory requirements, including the requirement that medicaid beneficiaries be given freedom of choice of their health care providers. In Arizona, there is an important experiment with competitive bidding to award state contracts for providers serving the medicaid population. In California, the strategy of regulated competition has resulted in two innovative legislative measures. First, beneficiaries of Medi-Cal (the California medicaid program) will be reimbursed only in designated hospitals that have received contracts to serve this population. Second, private insurers are now authorized to negotiate discounted reimbursement rates with providers, including competing economic units such as the emerging "Preferred Provider Organizations" (PPOs).

The challenge for policymakers pursuing a strategy of regulated competition is to design innovative rules and, in general, to create conditions in which market incentives can serve policy goals. The essential problem in these circumstances is how to avoid the stalemate that looms when proponents of the competition strategy ignore the limitations of the market mechanism and when the advocates of the regulation strategy appear to be responding more to the reality of market failure than to the possibilities of regulatory success.

ON LINKING HEALTH PLANNING AND FINANCING

Once it is realized that the regulation-competition dichotomy is misleading and that the competition strategy is more attractive than realistic, the current policy debate in America will no longer focus on the ideological questions of *whether* to regulate and *whether* to plan but on the more substantive questions of *how* to regulate and *how* to plan health care services to achieve implementation of health policy goals.

The case studies of France, Québec, and England, and

the preceding evaluation of health planning efforts in the United States suggest that in order to achieve implementation, it will be critical to link health planning and financing. Thus, in the future, whether a strategy of regulation or one of regulated competition is adopted, there are likely to be efforts at forging links between health planning activities in the DHSS, HSAs, SHCCs, SHPDAs, and those institutions responsible for provider reimbursement, health care budgeting, and actual service provision.

There is ample evidence in the United States that the existing reimbursement structure works at cross-purposes with health planning goals by encouraging costly institutional care, growth of specialized services, and excessive use of costly technology.[39] In linking health planning and financing, the challenge for policymakers will be to design both administrative and market incentives so that the behavior of physicians, hospitals, health plan competitors, and consumers conforms to cost containment goals. The problems this will entail confirm the risks of reposing more than limited faith either in facile models of unfettered competition or in heavy-handed regulation.

With regard to physicians, for example, linkage between health planning and financing would involve devising reimbursement incentives that influence the behavior of doctors in ways consistent with cost effective health enhancement goals. With regard to hospitals, it would involve the coordination of planning, rate setting, utilization review activities, and third party financing mechanisms in order to devise consistent policies that influence hospitals to make parsimonious use of technology-intensive services and to move in the direction of community medicine, preventive medicine, and occupational and social service programs. Finally, with regard to consumers and potential health plan competitors, linkage would involve the design of reimbursement incentives, voucher systems, rules and monitoring systems to ensure accurate information about proposed benefit packages and the quality of medical services actually provided. Let us review each of these "policy targets" in turn to elucidate the kinds of issues that efforts at linkage would be likely to raise.

LINKS TO PHYSICIAN REIMBURSEMENT

Although tampering with physician reimbursement provokes conflict between the medical profession and the state, the odds are that such intervention will continue and grow more politically explosive. Current methods of physician remuneration range from salary payment as in French and English public hospitals, to capitation payment as in the case of English GPs, to fee-for-service payment, the predominant method in Québec and in the United States. A strategy of regulated competition would create incentives for the development of HMO-type organizations that remunerate physicians on the basis of salary payment and possible bonuses. More likely, however, given the commitment of the American medical profession to fee-for-service payment, would be a strategy of regulation in which physicians are remunerated on a fee-for-service basis according to national or state fee schedules. Instead of reimbursing physicians under the prevailing "usual, customary, and reasonable" (UCR) fee structure used by Medicare, certain Medicaid programs, Blue Cross and Blue Shield plans, a national fee schedule would impose a list of maximum allowable reimbursements for specific medical procedures. As Robert Derzon, a former administrator of the Health Care Financing Administration observed, "Such schedules could be set either unilaterally by the government or by negotiations between government and physicians, but certainly not unilaterally by physicians."[40]

In principle, a national fee schedule could serve as an important administrative incentive for influencing physician behavior in directions consistent with health planning goals. Further, the determination of relative values of physician procedures would incorporate market incentives to influence physician behavior. In practice, however, there are problems in making fee schedules serve explicit goals.

Fee schedules are usually composed of two parts: coefficients that express the relative value of medical procedures and a conversion factor that translates the coefficient into a monetary value. Assuming perfect competition and constant returns to scale, conventional price theory would suggest that to promote efficiency, the coefficients should reflect relative costs. Thus, the price of each medical procedure would be set equal to its marginal cost. But since changes in both relative values and in the value of the multiplier are the subject of a bargaining process between a monopoly (the medical profession) and a monopsony (the state), price theory becomes a less helpful guide. Fee setting in such a context leads to a classic bilateral monopoly situation that, in traditional economic theory, has no determinate solution; that is, the resulting fees are determined more by skill in bargaining and, above all, by power—all of which are exogenous to the economist's preoccupations.[41]

Given the context of fee setting, it should not be surprising that physician fee schedules do not automatically produce incentives for achieving health planning goals. Since they reflect the relative bargaining power of professional specialty associations, they perpetuate built-in price distortions and inefficiency. For example, in France the value of a surgical procedure is constant regardless of whether it is performed by a general practitioner, a qualified surgeon, or a cardiologist and regardless of the presence and degree of preoperative or postoperative complications. As for consultations and home visits, their rate of reimbursement is constant regardless of whether the doctor spends five minutes or an hour, thus encouraging "fast medicine" and the multiplication of procedures. Finally, there is potentially the problem of price rigidity in most fee schedules: the relative values are not adjusted annually to account for such changes in technology as economies of scale in the production of laboratory tests or the introduction of microprocessors that reduce the unit cost of radiological equipment.

Whatever is decided with regard to a national fee schedule, to link health planning and physician reimbursement a number of important issues will have to be faced. Above all, it will be necessary to decide the extent to which fees should reflect the relative costs of producing services and the extent to which they should take account of broader planning goals, such as the pattern of physician location and specialty distribution. In addition, questions will undoubtedly arise about alternative criteria for guiding fee negotiations and about whether and, if so, to what extent fee-for-service payment should be replaced by prepaid forms of physician remuneration.

Links to Hospital Reimbursement

As with physician reimbursement, hospital reimbursement is also likely to undergo reform. Current methods for paying the hospital range from the cost-based system of reimbursement in France and the United States to systems of prospective annual budgets as in Québec and England.

A strategy of regulated competition is more likely to promote links with consumers and health plan competitors, whereas a strategy of regulation would focus on improving links between health planning activities and hospital reimbursement. As part of a broad strategy of regulation, several states have already legislated some form of hospital rate review and fostered institutional links between health planning agencies and rate review bodies. In Rhode Island, for example, a partnership was formed between planners and rate setters to promote common objectives within a limit on hospital spending—the maxicap model.[42] In Maryland, as early as 1968, the Health Services Cost Review Commission was the first agency to attempt regulation of hospitals, following the method used for public utilities, while encouraging comprehensive health planning agencies to develop a state plan.[43] Finally, in Massachusetts, New Jersey, New York, and Washington, various kinds of institutional linkage have been achieved.[44]

A pioneering experience in linking planning goals to hospital reimbursement is now in progress in New Jersey.[45] The State Department of Health, in collaboration with all third-party payers and the state hospital association, has agreed to link reimbursement directly to standardized costs identified by analysis of case mix as measured by diagnosis related groups (DRGs) and their average resource requirements. The most innovative aspect of this experiment is the establishment of a common language between doctors and administrators. In theory, this could enable health planners to identify patterns of resource consumption for similar medical conditions and to allocate hospital budgets accordingly.

Another approach to linkage focuses on a range of market incentives by third-party payers—for example, writing conformance clauses into Blue Cross plan contracts with providers and developing innovative payment mechanisms to stimulate elimination of excess capacity.[46] Such actions may involve reimbursement based on optimum utilization rates, reimbursement for fixed costs associated with closure of unneeded facilities, and limits on capital spending.

In contrast, still other advocates of linkage recommend administrative incentives, such as ceilings for regional health expenditures, thereby forcing explicit trade-offs not only for capital investments but for expenditures as well.[47] Indeed, the Carter administration's Hospital Cost Containment Bill proposed a national limit on capital spending and operating cost increases by hospitals.

In addition to institutional links, market incentives by third-party payers, and ceilings on regional health expenditures, linkage could potentially encourage cost effective modes of treatment and create disincentives for volume increases of hospital-based care and incentives for primary care, particularly in designated areas of need. Finally, linkage could be used as a mechanism for creating pooled depreciation funds out of which to allocate future investments in health infrastructure and perhaps even as a tool of health promotion strategies.

Whatever approaches are adopted by states to improve links between health planning activities and hospital reimbursement, a number of important organizational and technical questions will have to be addressed. To what extent should hospital reimbursement mechanisms incorporate the criteria developed by health planning agencies? Should rate setting and planning functions be combined and placed under a single agency such as a department of health, or should voluntary arrangements be established between rate-setting and planning agencies? Finally, from the perspective of provider reimbursement, should the rates of different payers—Medicare, Medicaid, Blue Cross, commercial insurance companies, out-of-pocket payers, and public organizations—be uniform? And if so, should the principal unit of reimbursement continue to be the hospital day or should measures of case mix such as DRGs be relied upon as in New Jersey?

LINKS TO CONSUMERS AND HEALTH PLAN COMPETITORS

A strategy of regulated competition must, almost by definition, concern itself with influencing the behavior of consumers as well as health plan competitors. Indeed, the essence of Enthoven's competition strategy is to create incentives for consumers to make conscious trade-offs between their premium rates and the scope and terms (coinsurance or deductibles) of services available to them and, also, to place providers at financial risk for inefficient organization and the provision of excessive services.

What might such an effort entail? Probably no less than a major health planning and perhaps even a national policing system to assure that health planning goals are properly linked to a system of market incentives for consumers and health plan competitors. Policymakers and planners would have to formulate and test the repercussions of alternative rules and regulations before designing them so as to achieve socially agreed-upon objectives. Regulators would have to design elaborate rules to ensure open enrollment periods, appropriate benefit packages, and fair marketing practices. Some new institutions, or changes in existing institutions, might be needed to assure conventional accreditation functions for health providers. Government antitrust specialists would have to police programs to ensure a vigorous and competitive economy within the health sector. Perhaps even a new profession of inspectors might emerge. In addition, an appropriate system of penalties would need to be developed for those institutions not abiding by the new rules of market competition.

It is hardly an exaggeration to suggest that a strategy of regulated competition would require the help of all the professionals currently working in the formal health planning establishment in America. No doubt, many of the tasks would need to be redefined. The rhetoric could easily be adjusted. For example, the Bureau of Health Planning could be called the "Bureau to Promote Competition in Health Care," and HSAs could be used to foster "fair competition" in their service areas. But even if such measures were adopted to provide proper incentives for consumers and providers, implementation of a regulated competition strategy would require tampering with powerful social forces.

On the demand side, as Enthoven has taken pains to explain, his health plan requires an end to the government's implicit policy of encouraging the growth of private health insurance. Since current federal tax provisions enable employers to deduct all their expenditures on health insurance for their employees, expensive health insurance plans receive higher subsidies than low cost ones. In addition, a worker in the 30 to 40 percent income tax bracket is better off getting sixty-five to seventy-five cents of desired services from another dollar of company-paid health insurance than adding that dollar to the amount of his taxable pay. The effects of such incentives, however, must be reexamined with respect not only to efficiency criteria but also to equity criteria. A major reason the incentives are there is because of past efforts by labor unions to extend health insurance coverage.[48] Enthoven proposes to get rid of such "goodies," but to drop the federal tax provisions would constitute a major intrusion into collective bargaining and would be sure to provoke resistance from labor and management.

On the supply side, there are also powerful forces that go against the rational proposal to create competing economic units that place health care providers at financial risk. The American Medical Association, for example, has not endorsed any of the procompetition bills currently before Congress. The American Hospital Association has endorsed the general principle, but the industry as a whole remains divided. It is not surprising that like other planning efforts to achieve significant change in the health sector, a strategy of regulated competition is likely to confront similar barriers to implementation.

Under the Reagan administration there has been a reaction against the growth of government programs in health. Cutbacks in Medicaid and Medicare will shift responsibilities from the federal government to state and local governments.[49] But simply shifting the financial burden downward will provide only temporary relief to Congress and state legislatures. Voluntary efforts at cost control combined with political rhetoric about the virtues of competition may slow down the growth of state intervention in the health sector and delay the imposition of tougher government controls. At some point, however—for better or for worse— stronger government controls, ranging from those now operating in France to those in Québec and England, are likely to be imposed in the United States.[50]

9
COMPARISONS AND
INTERPRETATIONS

We have examined the health planning predicament con-
ceptually and empirically, first in the background and approach to this study (Part II) and then in the case studies
(Part III). We have also evaluated, in retrospect, the experience with health planning in the United States. This chapter, the final one, summarizes what health planners have
done and particularly what they have failed to do. It begins
by reviewing two phases in the evolution of health planning
efforts—expansion and containment. Next, it highlights
the kinds of health planning distinguished in the case
studies and the problems of linking health planning and
health care financing. Most important, perhaps, this chapter considers three reasons advanced by scholars to explain
why health plans are so difficult to implement. The explanations are partial. They betray weaknesses. Nonetheless,
their effect is to reinforce the evidence about the difficulties
that health planners confront.

What are the prospects for health planning? The last
section of this chapter identifies three trends that shed light
on this question. One is the shift of public concern from
disease to health and the problems this raises in planning
for the social and environmental aspects of disease. The
second involves the management problems likely to accom-
pany the regionalization of health and social services. Fi-

nally, there is the shift of emphasis in health planning from a means of setting standards and augmenting resources to a means of distributing or rationing them. Each of these trends enlarges the scope of health planning. Each is sure to generate pressures to devise acceptable criteria for deciding who ought to have access to different services and under what conditions. Together, these trends are likely to intensify the sociopolitical conflicts now prevalent in the field of health planning and to provoke new ones.

EXPANSION AND CONTAINMENT

Two common phases may be distinguished in the evolution of health planning: (1) an expansionary phase characterized by planning efforts to improve access to health services and coordinate health sector growth and, (2) a containment phase characterized by planning efforts to control rising health care costs and to redistribute health resources within the health sector.

THE EXPANSIONARY PHASE

During the first phase, which lasted through the late sixties, most industrially advanced nations increased the health benefits for a majority of their population and successfully expanded and modernized their hospital infrastructure. The expansionary phase coincided with a fundamental belief in the medical paradigm—the potential of "scientific" medicine and modern technology to eradicate disease once and for all. Moreover, there was an implicit consensus that more is better. Subsidies for health resources development and biomedical research were expanded, and the responsibilities of medicine gradually grew to cover not only that portion of the population that came directly to seek care but also those who were ill but did not seek help.

On the demand side, the growth of the health sector was

fueled by massive infusions of public funds that significantly reduced the financial barriers to medical care.

In France, the national health insurance program, originally passed in 1928, was progressively extended until by 1960, 75 percent of the population was covered. Subsequently, coverage was extended to agricultural workers (1961), then to the self-employed (1965), and in 1978 to virtually the entire population, including the clergy.

In Québec, hospital insurance legislation was passed in 1961 and extended to ambulatory care in 1970. In England, universal coverage was achieved almost immediately with the creation of the National Health Service in 1948.

In the United States, Medicare and Medicaid legislation was passed in 1965 to provide national health insurance for the elderly and the poor. Although universal coverage has still not been achieved, the large majority of the population is now insured against the risk of hospitalization either through public or private health insurance.

On the supply side, state intervention in the health sector emphasized modernization and new construction of hospital infrastructure as well as subsidies for biomedical research.

In France, state policies aimed at reorganizing the supply of health services focused on hospital construction and reform. Passed in 1958, the Hospital Reform Act merged the best-equipped regional hospital facilities with teaching hospitals and initiated a gradual shift in reimbursement of hospital-based physicians from fee-for-service to salaries. The effect of this legislation was to modernize hospitals and consolidate the position of high technology medicine. By the late 1960s, France's public hospital infrastructure had been successfully modernized, and private cliniques had grown to include one-third of total acute care beds by the early 1970s.

In Québec the Hospitals Act was passed, in 1962, requiring legislative authorization for all hospitals and administrative compliance with provincial regulatory authorities. Following this legislation, public hospitals grew as former religious institutions were gradually financed by the provincial government.

In England, immediately following the creation of the NHS, supply-side policy also focused on hospital modernization. Although during the first seven years of the NHS only one new hospital was built, in 1962, while Enoch Powell was minister of health, a ten-year plan for balanced hospital development was produced. Its effect was not merely to promote hospital expansion but to replace small rural hospitals with modern district hospitals.

In the United States, the Hill-Burton Hospital Survey and Construction Act of 1946 provided federal aid to states for subsidizing the construction and modernization of hospital facilities in the private sector. In addition, in 1965, the Heart Disease, Cancer, and Stroke Amendments created Regional Medical Programs in fifty-six regions in order to speed up the application of biomedical knowledge by establishing cooperative arrangements among health care institutions, medical schools, and research centers.

THE CONTAINMENT PHASE

During the second phase in the evolution of health planning efforts, which began in the early seventies, there was an ideological shift regarding health policy and the role of the state. The faith in technological progress so characteristic of the expansionary phase dwindled. Policymakers shifted their emphasis from planning for hospital construction and modernization. They began designing cost containment policies and advocating demedicalization of health institutions and state intervention outside the medical sector to influence the social components of health.

Efforts to develop preventive health programs and "health promotion" campaigns, however, now carry overtones of victim blaming. Health professionals, particularly physicians, are subject to unsparing criticism while self-care and health promotion are proposed as a reaction to the growth of specialized medical services and technical procedures. Consumers are being urged to rediscover the virtues of self-reliance. In France, the national association of employers—the CNPF—is urging the need to *"responsabiliser les gens,"*[1] a recent task force in Québec urges major programs in occupational health and social services, and the English Consultative Document on Priorities emphasizes the importance of community care.[2] Aaron Wildavsky sums up this new ideology in the United States as follows: "Mother was right! You should eat a good breakfast everyday; you shouldn't smoke and you shouldn't drink; you should sleep seven or eight hours a day and not four or fourteen; and you shouldn't worry because it's bad for you."[3]

In order to control rising health care costs and redistribute health resources, health planners are increasingly preoccupied with the task of regulating the demand, the supply, and the distribution of health resources. They are designing incentives to promote the substitution of ambulatory for hospital care. They are also attempting to impose controls on hospital expansion and capital expenditures to reduce excess capacity and improve access to medical services. Planners are also calling for reimbursement and quality controls on hospitals and physicians. They are urging changes in methods of provider reimbursement from fee-for-service to capitation or prepaid systems in which physicians are encouraged to work on a salaried basis, to share in the risk of overspending, and to emphasize health maintenance. Finally, legislation has been passed and regulations have been devised to set national health priorities and establish national and regional health planning machinery.

In France since 1960, health care costs have risen at an even faster rate than in the United States. The legislative response to this situation was the Hospital Law of 1970, which sought to improve management in the public sector, control the unrestrained growth of the private sector, and promote a "harmonious" distribution of health services. In 1973 a national commission was charged with producing a national health plan. In addition, two regional commissions in each of France's twenty-one administrative regions were established to plan for health service needs and authorize construction of new cliniques or extensions of existing ones in the private sector.

In Québec, with the passage of Bill 42 in 1970, the Ministry of Health and the Ministry of the Family and Social Welfare were merged into the new Ministry of Social Affairs, which was charged with setting priorities, planning, programming, and evaluating. In 1971, with the passage of Bill 65, twelve regional councils (CRSSS) were created to determine health and social service needs of the population, prepare regional health plans, and coordinate investments in health sector infrastructure, particularly with regard to the newly created CLSCs. In addition, Castonguay, the minister of health, suspended a large number of ongoing hospital construction projects to channel the funds into domiciliary-care programs, CLSCs, and other programs in social medicine.

In England, with the administrative reorganization of the NHS in 1974, DHSS policymakers sought to eliminate the fragmentation of the former tripartite structure and to improve coordination by linking health services provided by the NHS with the social services provided by local authorities. In addition, by streamlining management functions and instituting a formal planning system, they sought to increase central control over resource allocation decisions.

Finally, in the United States, with the passage of the National Health Planning and Resources Development Act, a network of health planning agencies was established at area and state levels to produce annual and long-term health plans and to regulate hospital expansion and capital expenditures (see chap. 8).

RATIONALIZATION AND LINKAGE

In the case study of France two kinds of health planning were distinguished: (1) hospital construction and modernization, and (2) rationalization. Both kinds of planning occurred in Québec, England, and the United States, as well. In all these countries the state's intervention in the health sector promoted the construction and modernization of hospitals. Subsequently, health planners turned their attention to the problems of rationalizing the allocation of health resources. In Québec, health planning as social change and health planning as legislative reform are examples of rationalization. In England, health planning as reorganization and health planning as resource allocation are also attempts to rationalize the health sector. In the United States health planning as a strategy of decentralized state intervention is yet another form of rationalization policy.

Health planning as hospital construction and modernization succeeded admirably. But health planning as rationalization has encountered formidable barriers to implementation. The reasons for this lie in what health planners seek to accomplish and the institutional and historical context in which they operate. While hospitals were being built and modernized, there was widespread agreement on goals and a coalition of professional interests in favor of them. In contrast, while health planning efforts have focused on rationalization, there has been disagreement about goals and fewer means to pursue them.

France's struggle with rationalization has focused on efforts to control rising health care costs. It is a magnificent illustration of the health planning predicament. Since 1960 large injections of collective financing in combination with la médecine libérale have sent health care costs soaring. As early as 1969, a National Task Force challenged the notion of hospital-centered medical care, and deplored the dominant emphasis on "therapeutic engineering" techniques and the neglect of environmental and social aspects of illness. It advocated instead a regional health system that would encourage the substitution of ambulatory for inpatient hospital care. But the financial incentives underlying the French health system appear to work at cross-purposes with the guidelines promoted by health planners. The Hospital Law has not been implemented effectively; even the stopgap measures to achieve cost control have led to political stalemate.

As with France, the experience of Québec, England, and the United States suggests that health planners have been unable to alter significantly the allocation of health resources in conformance with health plans. In Québec, the Castonguay-Nepveu Commission succeeded in raising critical issues for public discussion. And the legislative reforms succeeded in significantly reorganizing the health sector. But there was no significant reallocation of resources. In England, although the 1974 reorganization succeeded in increasing centralization and managerial control, it has failed to unify effectively the tripartite structure. The Priorities Document and the RAWP Report are landmark efforts in specifying an equitable distribution of financial resources and tackling the problem of health care rationing. But they have so far failed to produce a consistent blueprint for allocating health resources and to influence those who decide the magnitude and distribution of budgetary allocations at the regional and subregional levels. Finally, in the United States, hospitals have been built and modernized, insurance coverage has grown, and a flexible, decentralized planning system has developed. The combination, however, of HSAs, SHPDAs, PSROs, HMOs and regulatory controls has failed to control the growth of health care costs and to reallocate health resources along the lines specified by state and local plans.

As noted in chapter 3, once links are improved between health planning activities and those institutions that finance health care, it should be possible for planners to design administrative and market incentives in such a way that the interests of health care providers converge, or at least do not work at cross-purposes with their goals. In practice, however, as we have seen in France, Québec, and England, the extent to which linkage can be achieved depends on the nature of resource allocation mechanisms—including provider reimbursement incentives—and on who controls this process.

In France, although financing for provider reimbursement is concentrated within the principal NHI Fund (the CNAMTS), there is, nevertheless, a failure to link health planning and financing. In Québec, where provider reimbursement and capital budgeting are centralized within the Ministry of Social Affairs, linkage of health planning and financing has been more effective—at least in containing the growth of the hospital sector. In England, although the Department of Health and Social Security controls both planning and financing, the tripartite administrative structure of the NHS has hindered coordination of policies on service development and the distribution of finance. The lesson of the English experience with health planning is that centralized control over financing and rationing of budgetary decisions may be necessary but not sufficient to link health planning criteria to the decision-making structure and thus alter the allocation of health resources.

As in France, Québec, and England, in the United States the problem of linking planning criteria to the institutions that control health care financing appears to be the Achilles' heel of contemporary health planning practice. Whether health planning strategies in the United States rely on regulation, competition, or regulated competition, sooner or later there is bound to be recognition that one strategy by itself cannot achieve appropriate linkages to health care financing. The issues raised by proposals to link health planning and financing suggest that strategies for health planning, like other efforts to bludgeon change in the health sector, are likely to encounter formidable barriers to implementation.

BARRIERS TO IMPLEMENTATION

Why is implementation of health planning goals so difficult to achieve? Explanations abound, but they are rarely convincing. A complete response to this question is not possible based on the case studies in this book. It is worthwhile, nevertheless, to examine three provocative views on the subject. Jean de Kervasdoué emphasizes the limited applicability of modern management techniques to problems in the health sector; Robert Alford proposes a theory of resistance by "structural interests" to explain stalemate in health care politics; and Marc Renaud stresses the systemic constraints to state intervention in the health sector, such as requirements of capital accumulation under capitalism.

Is it possible to make sense of such varied diagnoses? We shall attempt to do so by examining three questions: (1) Are health policy instruments adapted to medical practice? (2) Do structural interests in the health sector result in "dynamics without change"? (3) Are there structural constraints to state intervention?

ARE HEALTH POLICY INSTRUMENTS ADAPTED TO MEDICAL PRACTICE?

Jean de Kervasdoué suggests that health policies—in particular those that rely on regulatory instruments—are based on administrative technologies that were developed for industrial management.[4] Thus, concepts of health planning standards (e.g., hospital-bed/population ratios and management techniques such as cost-benefit analysis and quality control systems) are not adapted to medical practice. De Kervasdoué's hypothesis is that the barriers to implementation inhere in the policy instruments and approach, and this is why policymakers have difficulty controlling the health sector. De Kervasdoué implies that we would do better to understand the nature of the health system before proposing policy instruments to solve its problems. Can we conclude that an alternative set of policy instruments would succeed in implementing health policies and plans? If so, de Kervasdoué does not tell us what it is.

De Kervasdoué's hypothesis provides ammunition for analysts who subscribe to the conservative perspective on the proper role of the state in society. They would promptly agree that health policy instruments of a regulatory nature are not adapted to medical practice because problems in the health sector are misperceived, dramatized, and handled on the basis of the liberals' alleged conviction that "doing something" is equivalent to "doing good." Above all, analysts in this tradition emphasize the difficulties of implementation.

For example, Aaron Wildavsky conceives of a "theory of the political pathology of health policy."[5] This theory reviews all the classic dilemmas of policy planners who seek to solve "wicked problems," that is, problems that do not lend themselves to solutions because there is no "stopping rule" that allows for the final formulation of the problem.[6] But unlike de Kervasdoué, Wildavsky follows his analysis to the bitter end:

> Health policy is pathological because we are neurotic and insist on making our government psychotic. Our neurosis consists in knowing what is required for good health . . . and not being willing to follow this good advice. Government's ambivalence consists in paying, coming and going, once for telling people how to be healthy and once for paying their bills when they disregard this advice. Psychosis comes in when government persists in repeating this self-defeating play.[7]

In short, Wildavsky says, "We insist government do more, but when it does we like it less."[8] In Wildavsky's view we would be wise to have government do less.

De Kervasdoué would not necessarily support this conclusion. His main concern is not to provide a critique of state intervention but to elaborate his views on medical care system behavior. He explores the implications of a widely shared view in health economics—that our knowledge about production functions in health is primitive for two reasons: (1) there are no agreed-on measures of output (health); (2) there are multiple combinations of inputs that appear to produce the same output. De Kervasdoué does not expect the situation to change. His arguments are based on the view that "organizational technology [in medical care] is more ritualistic than rational, in the Weberian sense."[9]

De Kervasdoué stresses two points: (1) the technology of medical care, like that of education and the church, is justified not on the basis of empirically tested links between means and ends but on an a priori definition that may just as well be a function of moral or religious values as of past experience; and (2) policies to achieve greater equality of access to medical care and to control rising health care costs are based on arbitrary rules—administrative technologies, plans, policy instruments, and the like.

Because these rules focus on how resources ought to be allocated and prescribe imperfect measures to monitor the results, de Kervasdoué concludes that implementation is jeopardized from the start. The rules, however, are also influenced by the organizational strategies of actors within the health sector. What are these strategies? Who are the key actors? Unfortunately, aside from citing the work of Robert Alford, de Kervasdoué provides no further clues on these matters.

Do Structural Interests in the Health Sector Result in "Dynamics Without Change"?

Based on a study of efforts to plan and reform health care services in New York City, Robert Alford argues that there are significant barriers to implementation of health care reform and that the pluralistic interplay of health care politics must be understood in the context of a "battle—sometimes manifest, sometimes latent—of deeply embedded structural interests for control of key health care resources and institutions."[10] His term structural interest denotes three participants in health care politics. First, there are the "professional monopolists"—physicians both in private practice and in hospitals and medical schools, who share an interest in maintaining professional autonomy over their conditions of work. Second, there are the "corporate rationalizers"—health planners, hospital administrators, public health officials, and insurance companies, all of whom have an interest in extending the control of their institutions over the organization of medical care. Finally, there are the "equal health advocates"—the financially deprived interest groups that seek to increase responsiveness of the medical care system to their demands.

In Alford's theory, the professional monopolists represent "dominant interests," the corporate rationalizers are the "challenging interests," and the equal health advocates are the "repressed interests." The institutional and class structure of society sustains the power of the professional monopolists and the corporate rationalizers. What Alford calls "dynamics," the changing technology and division of labor in the production of health care, are likely to increase the power of the challenging interests and, therefore, the prospects for corporate rationalization of the health sector. According to this theory, "structural change," presumably the emancipation and triumph of the repressed interests, is needed but not likely to occur.

In one sense, this conclusion grows out of the liberal perspective on the role of the state in society. It is consistent with the conventional pluralist approach in political science, which explains social change in terms of small increments.[11] Within this framework, analysts focus on the marginal adjustments along a political equilibrium and are quick to identify the obstacles to significant change. For example, in the context of English health policy, Rudolf Klein argues that the growth of the health sector has led to the growing participation in policymaking of divergent interest groups— trade unions, associations of health professionals, Community Health Councils, and "particular client groups, ranging from the mentally ill and handicapped to psoriasis sufferers."[12] The result has been to multiply veto power, thus making decision making more costly and slower and creating a situation which Klein calls "corporate stalemate."

The pluralist approach, however, fails to distinguish group participation from group influence and the relative dominance of certain groups. This has resulted, as Theodore Lowi put it, in

> case-study after case-study that "proves" the model with find-ings directed by the approach itself. Issues are chosen for research because conflict made them public; group influence is found because in public conflict groups participate whether they are influential or not. Group influence can be attributed because they so often share in the *definition* of the issue and have taken positions that are more or less directly congruent with the outcomes. An indulged group was influential, and a deprived group was uninfluential; but that leaves no room for group irrelevancy.[13]

Turning to what is often called "dominant interest group theory," Roger Friedland suggests:

> Because of the intensity of their interests and the public indis-pensability of their politically enforced monopolies of skills, information, or specialized capital, . . . producer groups are usually able to dominate both political and administrative arenas where the substance of state intervention in social service delivery is actually determined.[14]

Similarly, Marmor, Wittman, and Heagy have distin-guished between "concentrated versus diffuse interests."[15] In the case of policies to control rising costs in the health sector, if implementation succeeds, the diffuse public would pay lower health insurance premiums and medical fees. Success is unlikely, however, because providers are bound to mobilize their concentrated interests to oppose such policies.

Although Alford's conclusions are consistent with those of pluralist analysts, his study falls clearly within the framework of dominant interest group theory:

> To summarize the argument in a nutshell, the "crisis" of health care is not a result of the necessary competition of diverse

interests, groups, and providers in a pluralistic and competitive health economy, nor is it a result of bureaucratic inefficiencies to be corrected by yet more layers of administration established by government policy. Rather the conflicts between the professional monopolists . . . and the corporate rationalizers . . . account for many of the aspects of health care summarized above. These conflicts stem, in turn, from a fundamental contradiction in modern health care between the character of the technology of health and the private appropriation of the power and resources involved. . . . Government is not an independent power standing above and beyond the competing interest groups, but represents changing coalitions of elements drawn from various structural interests.[16]

This summary of the essence of Alford's theory also reflects its weaknesses. Alford never goes beyond defining the structural interests and asserting that they "account for many aspects of health care summarized above," that is, the apparent stalemate or "dynamics without change."[17] He neither presumes to derive his theory from his case studies nor proposes any strategies to overcome the "barriers to reform." Are we to suppose that these barriers are insurmountable short of a "much more fundamental struggle to change American social institutions"?[18] If so, how is one to explain the profound changes that have already occurred in the health systems of Western industrial nations? And how would Alford explain the changes that occurred in the United States in passing from the expansion to the containment phase of health planning?

Alford makes an oblique reference to the "fundamental contradiction . . . between . . . the technology of health care and the private appropriation of power and resources involved."[19] But he never pursues this idea. He also makes a number of references to a theory of the state as a "changing coalition of elements drawn from the various structural interests."[20] Since he is generally sympathetic to interpretations that stem from the radical perspective on the role of the state, one would expect more analysis of the limits of state intervention in the health sector, but Alford does not develop this issue.

ARE THERE STRUCTURAL CONSTRAINTS TO STATE INTERVENTION?

Based on his study of health care reform in Québec, Marc Renaud argues that there are limits to state intervention and that these limits are defined by a structure: the capitalist mode of production.[21] In his view, under capitalism, only those health "needs" that can be transformed into commodities are recognized and satisfied in order to sustain capital accumulation. In a sense, such a view is tautological since capitalism may be defined as that mode of production that is characterized by substitution of exchange values for use values, that is, commodification. Nevertheless, Renaud provides insights for the analysis of health planning and policy:

> Beyond the most apparent and often nationally specific constraints, such as the existing institutional arrangements, the demands and pressures of interest groups, the electoral platforms of political parties, the national structure of political decision-making, and the inextricable problems of management and coordination embedded in a given health system, state interventions in the health field are bound everywhere in the capitalist world by less visible yet real constraints that are deeply rooted in the capitalist mode of production and that are largely above the volition of individual health care workers, public officials, and the citizenry alike. . . . The dominant engineering approach of contemporary scientific medicine equates healing and consumption, that is, in more general terms, health needs and the commodity form of their satisfaction, thus legitimating and facilitating capitalist economic growth despite its negative health consequences.[22]

With the term "negative health consequences," Renaud refers to iatrogenic effects of scientific medicine and to the social costs of industrialization. Why "capitalist economic growth" is any worse than socialist or any other kind of economic growth is not explained. Renaud moves on. In spite of increasing evidence of the limitations of modern medicine and of the growth of "diseases of civilization," he asks why countries invest between 5 and 10 percent of their GNP in curative medicine while public health and preventive medicine remain relatively neglected. His answer is that "the state [under capitalism] can only aggregate individual needs into national budgets and plans but it cannot reorganize the economy so that less illness is produced."[23] Why? Renaud relies largely on the work of analysts who share the radical perspective on the role of the state in capitalist society.

Like James O'Connor, Renaud proceeds on the premise that the "capitalist state must try to fulfill two basic and mutually contradictory functions—accumulation and legitimation."[24] Like Claus Offe, he accepts the notion of a "class based state" that "must at the same time practice its class character and keep it concealed."[25] For Renaud, the state, in dealing with the health sector, is caught in a "very precarious equilibrium" in which it must balance the economic requirements of the health industry with the demands of the public to improve the conditions of social harmony. This contradiction leads him to consider the "internal dynamics" of state intervention in health.

Renaud argues that the state may intervene in four directions in order to improve the health care system:

1. It may subsidize both the supply and demand of medical care. (Such interventions characterize what we have called the expansion phase of health planning.) Although such a strategy can lead to some redistribution of health resources, it never questions the logic of the existing institutions.[26]

2. It may blame individuals for their health problems. Such a strategy threatens neither the engineering model of medicine nor capital accumulation. It may even assist industries producing protective devices for occupational health programs and favor the development of new industries such as diet foods and exercise equipment.

3. It may regulate industries whose products might pollute, such as tobacco, food, and drugs. Such a strategy, however, is "self-defeatingly dependent upon economic growth to solve the problems associated with such growth."[27] Since this form of state intervention would threaten capital accumulation in some profitable economic sectors, it is unlikely to occur.

4. It may urge an entirely different approach to medicine, "the decommodification of health needs leading to a more direct and intense preoccupation with the social conditions giving rise to disease."[28] But this strategy would require the elimination of the medical profession's monopoly of the definition and cure of illness; the private appropriation of skills, training, and credentials; and the actual trends in the allocation of health resources. These are precisely the kinds of changes that are structurally constrained by the capitalist mode of production and "ultimately only possible in socialist societies."[29]

Whereas Alford's theory explains the stalemate resulting from the conflict between corporate rationalizers and professional monopolists, Renaud's theory goes farther and suggests that aside from structural interests there are limits beyond which even corporate rationalization cannot succeed in changing the structure of the health sector. His theory, however, is flawed in several respects. For example, Renaud assumes that diseases of civilization could be eliminated in a socialist society because "in theory" it would not be constrained by the pressures of commodifying the engineering model of medicine. Besides, it would "give precedence to human needs rather than to capital accumulation."[30] Such a view is romantic and surprising in light of his own admission that "it remains an open question whether the diseases of civilization are tied to industrialization *per se* or whether they are linked to the specifically capitalist mode of economic growth."[31]

Renaud never explains what, exactly, he means by the concept "capitalist mode of production." He does not resolve the ambiguity concerning problems related to industrialism versus those resulting from capitalism. Nor does he develop O'Connor's concepts of accumulation and legitimation and Offe's theories about the internal structure of the capitalist state. Drawing on Renaud's theory, for example, how would one explain why many capitalist countries pursue policies against the interests of accumulation in the tobacco industry? (We will overlook the fact that most self-proclaimed socialist countries have not engaged in anti-smoking campaigns.)

Such state intervention could be justified by invoking the concept of legitimacy; or one might qualify the accumulation impulse, as Renaud does, by specifying that state intervention must be compatible with capital accumulation as a whole, which is not necessarily "congruent with accumulation in specific industries." Such an explanation is too broad, however. Offe has developed more refined concepts to classify alternative mechanisms of state intervention within capitalist society, for example, "negative and positive selection mechanisms" that allow one to classify a range of possible state responses to particular problems.[32] But Renaud has not applied these concepts to the health sector. He leaves us only with the concept of structural constraints.

IMPLICATIONS FOR HEALTH PLANNING

The question of whether health policy instruments are adapted to medical practice prompted us to note how state intervention in the health sector is often self-defeating. The question of whether structural interests in the health sector result in "dynamics without change" led us to explore both pluralist and dominant interest group theories of social change. And the question of whether there are structural constraints to state intervention led us to consider theories of the capitalist state and the limitations of structural analysis.

The ideas generated by these questions and the responses to them are not mutually exclusive; quite the contrary. When they are combined, they provide compelling reasons for anticipating powerful barriers to implementation of health planning goals. These barriers are substantial—even though it is true that the insights discussed above are partial and the views developed do not lend themselves to decisive empirical tests.

EMERGING TRENDS

Health planners find themselves at the center of conflict when they propose policies that would promote social reform and alter the distribution of power. The conflict is unlikely to wither away. That is why, over the next decade, the questions of who should participate in health planning and whose interests health planners should serve will become sharper and inescapable—both at home and abroad.[33] These tendencies appear all the more likely if we examine the probable effects of three emerging trends: (1) the broadening goals of health systems; (2) the regionalization of health services; and (3) the advent of health care rationing.

THE BROADENING GOALS OF HEALTH SYSTEMS

As health planning has evolved from the expansion to the containment phase, health system goals have broadened rather than narrowed. Initially health systems sought to cure and care for that portion of the population that demanded health services—the exposed part of the so-called iceberg of disease. More recently, however, responsibility has been enlarged to include curing and caring for that part of the population that is ill but does not seek help—the submerged part of the iceberg of disease.[34] Epidemiologic studies carried out in diverse nations (Lévy et al. in France,

Wolfe in Canada, Last in England, and Bogatyrev in the Soviet Union) suggest that for most conditions the submerged part of the iceberg is much larger than the visible one.[35] As health system goals continue to broaden, the utilization of health services is likely to increase significantly. For example, health services will be provided not only to patients with heart disease but also to that portion of the population displaying such high risk factors as smoking, hypertension, and high cholesterol.

At the present time, health system goals are expanding to cover the social components of disease at individual and community levels: alcoholism, drug addiction, and juvenile delinquency. Among the new areas are vocational rehabilitation, marriage counseling, sex therapy, and treatment of mental or nervous disorders reflecting postindustrial stresses such as the accelerated rate of social and technical change, large displacements in commuting to and from work, and frequent migrations in the course of a lifetime. The emerging phase, in which most industrially advanced nations now find themselves, is the expansion of the traditional responsibility of a health system beyond that of caring for the submerged part of the iceberg of disease, beyond treatment of social pathologies, to its potential of assuring what the World Health Organization calls a "state of well being." In this sense, the pill as a contraceptive, a sedative, a hallucinogen, or an antihypertensive is a symbol of the search for more choice, more self-control, more inner coherence. These new health system goals are especially valued in a postindustrial society where traditional social networks, such as the family and the church, are eroding.[36]

To meet the broadening goals of health systems, health planners will have to intervene both inside and outside the medical sector. The Lalonde Report in Canada is the most celebrated document that recognized this point. But other countries have also followed suit, particularly in the area of prevention.[37] In France, the Ministry of Health has conducted major highway safety and anti-cigarette-smoking campaigns. It has also taken steps to increase day-care services for mothers and children. In England, there has been an important trend in the direction of new caring environments; for example, hospices for the dying and home-care programs. In Sweden, health planners have expanded their interest in occupational health from problems of safety and exposure to noxious substances to include the issues of worker and consumer satisfaction. Other industrially advanced nations are likely to follow this trend.

The improvement of consumer satisfaction usually implies more consumer participation. Consumers have grown reluctant to delegate responsibility exclusively to professionals either for their own care or for the management of health care institutions. Some even concur with George Bernard Shaw's sardonic dictum that every profession, and the medical profession in particular, is a "conspiracy against the laity."[38] This attitude has been most evident in the more community-oriented CLSCs in Québec. In England, despite the creation of community health councils, consumer participation has been less vociferous. And in France, although there is no precedent for consumer participation in public administration, trade unions have sometimes advocated consumer interests in addition to producer interests, particularly within the CNAMTS.

As health planners face broadening health system goals, at the national level they will have to articulate a broader concept of health and make judgments about social priorities. At the regional level, they will have to plan for social and environmental concepts of disease, not just for somatic health services.

THE REGIONALIZATION OF HEALTH SERVICES

Throughout the world in nations differing widely in social and economic systems, there is a trend toward regionalization of health services.[39] A regional hierarchy of health services is supposed to promote efficient resource allocation, reduce disparities in resource distribution, and improve the range and quality of health care.[40] Coupled with financial incentives, regionalization can redirect *demand* to the less expensive programs and facilities and provide the organizational leverage for extending and sharing limited health manpower and facilities.

In principle, a regional network, with decentralized resources in the periphery for primary and secondary care and with a center reserved for capital-intensive tertiary care, will balance several important aims—the quest for more consumer participation, better access, and the centralization required to achieve possible economies of scale in production and high quality of delivery. In practice, such a scheme raises some important problems. First, criteria for resource allocation must be generated. Second, useful geographic boundaries of regions must be established for planning. In addition, linkages must be assured between the various levels of care, such as referrals and information flow.

In addition to the situations in France, Québec, and England, there is evidence from other health systems in industrially advanced nations that the challenge of regionalization is being met in several ways. In Sweden, for example, regionalization was accepted in 1958 when Parliament approved the recommendations of the Royal Commission on Regionalization of Health Services. The country was divided into eight health regions, each with a population of one million. Six regional teaching hospitals were improved, and two new ones were planned in order to maximize accessibility to tertiary-care services. In addition, at subregional levels, each of Sweden's twenty-three county councils finances over one-half of health care expenditures and plays an important part in planning the structure of county health care organization.

In the Soviet Union, despite the centralized nature of health planning and severe disparities in the distribution of health resources between and within regions (*oblasts**),

*Soviet administrative regions with populations ranging from one to five million.

health services are, nevertheless, organized in a regional network.[41] Primary care physicians are organized by specialities through polyclinics in *uchastoks** and assigned responsibility for caring for the population in their districts and referring more serious cases to the secondary and tertiary levels. What is more, a network of *sanipeds* is organized within all oblasts to provide certain public health services and to gather epidemiologic data with which to service primary-care physicians. Most noteworthy is the transition from concern for the individual patient to concern for the health of a designated population at the regional level.

As the trend toward regionalization of health care continues, health services must increasingly be planned not only according to different categories of diagnostic, preventive, or therapeutic care and not only by physical, emotional, or social components of disease but also they must be planned according to level of care—primary, secondary, and tertiary—in which a range of services is functionally integrated. In this framework, the functional integration of health services consists of linking primary-care services to the tertiary level and tertiary care back to the primary level for rehabilitation and follow-up services. If regions acquire greater discretion over the financing of health care and if greater emphasis is placed on caring for the health of a target population than on caring for individuals who seek medical care, functional integration of health services is likely to increase, and regional health planning may then exercise greater control over the allocation of health resources.

THE ADVENT OF HEALTH CARE RATIONING

As health planning evolved from the expansionary phase to the containment phase, it also began to shift from an exercise in standard setting to a strategy for the explicit

*Microdistricts with populations ranging from 3,000 to 65,000.

rationing of health services in the context of budgetary constraints.[42] The shift from planning by standards to planning by rationing is more than a substitution of methods; it represents the transformation of health planning from a means of augmenting health resources to a means of distributing them. This shift also reflects a new concept of need—one that is concerned with deriving criteria for rationing health resources.

When standards were used as the principal technique of identifying health needs, health planners were remarkably successful in justifying the development of new services and the expansion of existing ones. Indeed, nineteenth-century social reformers used this concept of need to establish engineering codes and government standards for public hygiene. Twentieth-century physicians used it to establish minimal levels of competence in scientific medicine. Both groups invoked what has been called *normative need*: professionally set norms focusing on service inputs.[43] Thus, while standards became the guardians of quality and the predominant tool of health planning, they insulated the social reformers from the radical's challenge of participation and protected the turf of the medical profession from encroachment by competing groups of healers.[44]

In contrast, rationing makes these trade-offs transparent, for it forces health planners to set goals and to use them as explicit criteria by which to decide who ought to have access to what services under what conditions and at what cost. Rationing may occur at the clinical, institutional, regional, or national level—or at all of them.[45] On the supply side, planners can ration health care by modifying the organization, quantity, and distribution of manpower, beds, and equipment, as well as by affecting provider behavior through reimbursement incentives and regulatory mechanisms. On the demand side, planners can ration health care by affecting utilization through pricing policies—both money and time—and through primary, secondary, or tertiary prevention to reduce potential need for acute services.

Although rationing has always been an implicit part of health planning, explicit rationing is only now beginning to emerge. In France, on the supply side, health planners have limited the growth of new hospitals, have developed a review process for capital expenditures, have imposed new restrictions on the number of medical school graduates, and currently plan to finance public hospitals on the basis of prospective annual budgets. On the demand side, the CNAMTS has maintained a copayment for ambulatory care and is now considering restricting the extent of coverage for certain services.

In Québec, supply-side rationing is more decentralized and occurs at the level of the individual institution through closed-budget systems for hospitals and CLSCs. On the demand side, although all medical services are free at the point of consumption, Québec has aggressively developed preventive health and social services. To date, Québec, unlike France, has partially formulated a coherent strategy for rationing health resources. In contrast, English health planners have exercised central control over capital expenditures and supply-side rationing of financial resources since the creation of the NHS in 1948. But it is only since the emergence of health planning as resource allocation in the mid-1970s (e.g., the Priorities Document and RAWP) that the consequences of rationing decisions have been examined and explicit criteria have been developed to guide this process. Demand-side rationing in the form of queues operates for some services, notably elective surgery and ambulatory specialty care. Queuing, however, appears to have been less of an explicit rationing strategy than a miscalculation on the part of NHS planners about the relativity of need for medical care.[46]

The emergence of explicit rationing has three principal implications for health planning practice. First, health planners will have to begin thinking about planning under more severe resource constraints. They will have to weigh the relative importance of health as opposed to other social goals. And this process will have to occur at national, regional, and local levels.

Second, health planners will increasingly be called on to reformulate broad system goals into criteria for achieving efficient resource allocation and equitable distribution of health resources. Standards—the traditional resource allocators—appear destined to be replaced by new rationing criteria using output-oriented indicators such as health status indices. Traditional service units such as obstetrics or coronary care will give way to planning for broader categories such as fertility-related care and cardiovascular diseases, thus permitting substitution of service inputs and trade-offs between preventive, curative, rehabilitative, or caring services, and levels of care.

Third, health planners will have to monitor and evaluate the effects of health expenditures on societal values—not just on health status and on health system goals. In considering explicit methods of rationing, health planners will be increasingly pressed to examine the implications of such concepts as individual liberty, pluralism, and social choice in light of the political institutions and historic responses to these issues within specific nations.

Appendix 1
COMPARATIVE HEALTH SYSTEMS: NOTES ON THE LITERATURE

Comparative research on health systems has largely ignored the health planning predicament.[1] It has focused on describing the organization of medical care and explaining variation on the basis of received theories within such disciplines as anthropology, sociology, political science, and economics.[2] Historically, three stages of comparative health systems research may be distinguished.[3] During the first stage, which dominated until the mid-sixties, travelogues were written by physicians returning from exotic tours.[4] This tradition is still present in various medical journals.[5] During the second stage—still flourishing today—medical care systems were described from several points of view. For example, Milton Roemer's essays on aspects of health system organization around the world; John Fry's book on the medical care system in the Soviet Union, the United States, and the United Kingdom; Douglas-Wilson and McLachlan's collection of papers on international health prospects; Fry and Farndale's collection on comparative medical care organization; and Victor and Ruth Sidel's vignettes of the health care system in Sweden, Great Britain, the Soviet

Union, and China.[6] In addition, some case studies were produced. For example, Gordon Forsyth and Almont Lindsey on England, Victor and Ruth Sidel on China, Gordon Hyde and Henry Sigerist on the Soviet Union, and Richard Weinerman on Eastern Europe.[7] During the third stage, which we are now entering, there is an attempt to make the field of comparative health systems into a kind of social science.

The social science approach to comparative health systems has the inherent defects of its virtues. On the one hand, it has assembled relevant descriptive materials, classified them, elaborated hypotheses, and tested them against available evidence. On the other hand, to achieve a rigorous study design, the social science approach has often focused on the more static cross-sectional comparisons of health systems and has, of necessity, narrowed significantly the scope of research questions. To date, Kohn and White's international collaborative study on the determinants of medical care utilization and Robert Maxwell's comparative analysis of health care expenditures are probably the most sophisticated examples of this approach.[8]

Although a number of excellent case studies have been produced during the third stage of comparative health systems research (e.g., Harry Eckstein, Derek Gill, and Vicente Navarro, on England; Christa Altenstetter and Deborah Stone, on Germany; and Mark Field and Vicente Navarro, on the Soviet Union),[9] this stage is also characterized by the erosion of ideals shared by stage-two scholars, who were motivated by the practical concerns of improving the social organization of medical care. Their ideals have often been superseded by those of scholars who show more interest in the theoretical concerns of social science justice. The social science approach to comparative health systems has raised a number of important methodological and conceptual issues and generated some provocative cross-national studies related to convergence and divergence of medical care organization in industrially advanced nations.

METHODOLOGICAL ISSUES

The fundamental methodological issue in comparative health systems research involves devising a study design and selecting alternative systems that allow the analyst to hold some variables constant while manipulating experimental ones. In the area of health policy, for example, how does one evaluate the success of cost containment efforts in health systems characterized by diverse patterns of financing and provider reimbursement? Quasi-experimental research designs would suggest matching two health systems on all but a few policy-related factors. But "matching," let alone a real experiment, is rarely feasible in health systems research.

One response to this difficulty has been to match health systems on at least some criteria (e.g., levels of health resources), and then to call for "in-depth studies of contrasting cases."[10] Another response has been to use the language of natural experiment and view "most similar systems" as laboratories in which to assess the effects of alternative policy options at home.[11] This study has combined both approaches, that is, has presented case studies of similar systems.

Another methodological concern in the social science approach to comparative health systems research is whether the descriptive studies and data collected during stage two are actually comparable. If they are not, this casts great doubt on the utility of making international comparisons. If they are, qualifications must usually be made. Indeed, during stage three, there have been more papers devoted to making the requisite methodological qualifications than to actual cross-national studies.[12]

The most difficult methodological issues arise in evaluating health systems, for this involves specifying the relationship between the elements of a health system (inputs) and their impact on health (output). But how does one distin-

guish the impact of health services on health from the
impacts of improvements in social services, economic security, education, transportation—not to mention the social
and physical environment? This problem raises the issue of
measurement techniques such as health status indicators. It
also explains why, in his comparative study of the United
States, Sweden, and England, Odin Anderson found it
impossible to attribute differences in the usual health
indices of morbidity and mortality to patterns of medical
care organization in these countries.[13] To evaluate health
systems, it is necessary to agree on consistent definitions of
health system inputs and to devise health status indicators to
measure outputs. Such considerations raise a number of
conceptual issues.

CONCEPTUAL ISSUES

The concept of health system is clearly central. And yet
there is no fully satisfactory definition of this concept, for it
is difficult to agree both on the boundaries of the system and
on a definition of health. Henrik Blum provides a visual
model of health, suggesting that health care services are
merely one input into health among three others—hered-
ity, behavior, and environment (fig. 15). Richard Weinerman, one of the first scholars to advance the social science
approach to comparative health systems, defines the health
system as "all of the activities of a society which are designed
to protect or restore health, whether directed to the individual, the community, or the environment."[14] Odin
Anderson has more concretely outlined the "boundaries of
a relatively easily defined system with entry and exit points,
hierarchies of personnel, types of patients"—in short, what
he calls "the officially and professionally recognized 'helping' services regarding disease, disability, and death."[15]
    Viewing the concept of health system at a macrosociolog-
ical level, Mark Field proposes the following formal definition: "that societal mechanism that transforms generalized

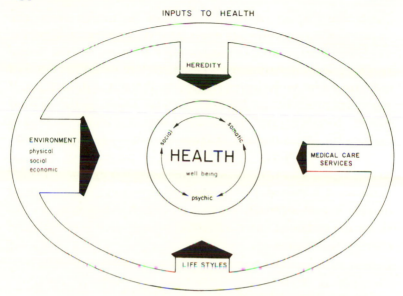

Fig. 15. Inputs to health.

Source: Adapted from H. Blum, *Planning for Health*, 2nd ed. (New York: Human
Sciences Press, 1981), p. 3.

resources into specialized outputs in the form of health
services." He adds that "the 'health system' of any society is
that social mechanism that has arisen or been devised to deal
with the incapacitating aspects of illness, trauma, and (to
some degree) premature mortality . . . the five D's: death,
disease, disability, discomfort, dissatisfaction."[16]

Another approach to the concept of health system is to
define it implicitly by postulating a causal model of it. Thus,
drawing on Ray Elling's proposed framework for studying
health systems, De Miguel outlines four subsystem levels
that influence health status: individual, institutional, societal, and environmental.[17] Such an approach allows one to
analyze a health system by investigating the effects of a
hierarchy of independent variables on the dependent var-
iable, health status. It also raises questions about the most
effective levels at which to effect system change.

CONVERGENCE VERSUS DIVERGENCE

In addition to the methodological and conceptual issues, the social science approach to comparing health systems has led some scholars to emphasize the convergent evolution of health systems and others to emphasize their divergent sociopolitical contexts and patterns of organization.

Among the convergence theorists, David Mechanic and Mark Field have written convincing briefs based on their cross-national studies of health systems. In a concise review of comparative health systems research, Mechanic argues that the growth of biomedical knowledge and medical technology has had such a pervasive impact on the shape of health care delivery systems that countries with different ideological preferences have had to confront common problems.

> The hypothesis of convergence does not imply that medical systems, which develop out of the particular historical and cultural background of a nation and its dominant ethos, will not continue to have distinct characteristics reflecting the ideological orientations and the socio-cultural context of a country. But the basic pattern of practice in modern society is increasingly dominated by the imperatives of the emerging technology, the objective pattern of morbidity in the population, and the worldwide phenomenon of growing public expectations.[18]

In a study on differentiation and convergence in health systems, Field identifies five ideal-type health systems and argues that the direction of change in modern societies is moving from the system of type 1 to that of type 5 (table 11). Since these ideal types reflect the diversity of existing patterns of medical care organization, it is worth characterizing them briefly.

Type 1 is the *private health system*—one in which the physician works as an entrepreneur in office-based private practice and is remunerated on a fee-for-service basis. Type 2 is the *pluralistic health system*—one much like that of the United

TABLE 11
The Evolution of Health Systems

Health system	Type 1 Private	Type 2 Pluralistic	Type 3 National health insurance	Type 4 National health service	Type 5 Socialized health service
General definition	Health care as item of personal consumption	Health care as predominantly a consumer good or service	Health care as an insured/guaranteed consumer good or service	Health care as a state-supported consumer good or service	Health care as a state-provided public service
Position of the physician	Solo entrepreneur	Solo entrepreneur and member of variety of groups/organizations	Solo entrepreneur and member of medical organizations	Solo entrepreneur and member of medical organizations	State employee and member of medical organizations
Role of professional associations	Powerful	Very strong	Strong	Fairly strong	Weak or nonexistent
Ownership of facilities	Private	Private and public	Private and public	Mostly public	Entirely public
Economic transfers	Direct	Direct and indirect	Mostly indirect	Indirect	Entirely indirect
Prototypes	U.S.; Western Europe; Russia in 19th century	U.S. in 20th century	Sweden; France; Canada; Japan in 20th century	Great Britain in 20th century	Soviet Union in 20th century

Source: Adapted from M. Field, *Comparative Health Systems: Differentiation and Convergence*, Final Report, Grant #HS-00272 (Washington, D.C.: National Center for Health Services Research, 1978).

States today, where there is a wide range of organizational arrangements for providing medical care and where physicians are remunerated in a variety of ways: fee-for-service payment, capitation payment, prepayment, and salary. Type 3 is the *national health insurance system*—one that resembles the pluralistic system, except that there is concentrated financing; that is, most financial transfers are made via the state or a quasi-public agency such as Social Security. Type 4 is the *national health service system*—one where most facilities are owned by the state and where most physicians are remunerated on the basis of salaries and capitation fees. Type 5 is the *socialized health service*—one where all facilities are owned and managed by the state and where all employees are salaried by the state.

Field does not suggest that there will be eventual convergence. In spite of his structural-functional perspective, indeed, his Parsonian bent, he is quite prepared to recognize the importance of cultural diversity, historical specificity, and ideological and political differences among nations. But he sees these factors as adding "their own coloration to the world."[19] His principal argument is that the evolution of health systems in the direction of type 5

> seems in line with the changes one observes in modern (and modernizing) societies, e.g., such trends as increased internal differentiation of specialized units of society . . . a change from *Gemeinschaft* or traditional society to a *Gesellschaft* or an associational, businesslike, modern type of society; a change from informal groups to bureaucracies; a change in the direction of the increased application of rationality and calculability and hence predictability and planning.[20]

Among those scholars who have emphasized the divergent characteristics among health systems in industrially advanced nations, Milton Roemer and Theodore Marmor have urged cross-national comparisons to derive lessons for policymakers.[21] Victor Sidel has sought "inspiration in the efforts of other societies."[22] Others have argued that we have not yet developed adequate vocabulary to make meaningful comparisons.[23] Nevertheless, several thoughtful case studies and cross-national comparative studies have been produced, all of which focus on divergent aspects of health systems.

The more interesting case studies appear in books edited around specific themes. Banta and Kemp have edited a superb study on the management of medical technology in nine countries.[24] De Kervasdoué, Kimberly, and Rodwin have edited a study on the future of health policy in France, Québec, Britain, and the United States.[25] McLachlan and Maynard have edited a study of the interactions between public and private sectors in the delivery of health care services in Western Europe, the United States, Canada, and Australia.[26]

William Glaser has produced three cross-national comparative studies. The first attempts to explain the impact of the social structure on the organization of hospitals.[27] The second describes systems of physician remuneration and analyzes their effects on medical care organization.[28] And the third attempts to explain how alternative administrative arrangements affect the nature of the bargaining process between the medical profession and the state.[29]

In addition to Glaser's work, Brian Abel-Smith and John Babson have written general comparative studies on the evolution and current diversity of systems for health care financing and organization.[30] Blanpain, Delesie, and Nys have analyzed the development of health resources in five European countries.[31] Ake Blomqvist has examined the evidence on advantages and disadvantages of private versus public health care systems in the United States, the United Kingdom, and Canada.[32] Jozef Van Langendonck has written the most comprehensive study on the evolution and current administration of health insurance in Europe.[33] Robert Maxwell has studied patterns of health care organization in Western Europe, the United States, and the Soviet Union.[34]

Another approach to analyzing the divergent characteristics of health systems has been to compare differences in health care policies. Milton Roemer has done this for policies ranging from financing to regulation and to manpower issues; Odin Anderson underscores the extent to which health policy and the structure of health systems are rooted in their sociopolitical contexts; and Howard Leichter brings a political science perspective to the field.[35]

Leichter's book is noteworthy, for he provides an "accounting scheme" within which to analyze the determinants of health policies. Leichter applies this scheme to four case studies (Great Britain, Germany, Japan, and the Soviet Union) and provides plausible reasons for particular policies being followed in each country. Like Odin Anderson, however, he does not provide an evaluation of these policies. Further, along with Anderson, he does not analyze health planning efforts.

As far as I know, with the exception of some journal articles, a World Health Organization comparison of planning methods and two international conferences, there has been no cross-national study of health planning efforts.[36]

APPENDIX 2
ACRONYMS

France

CNAMTS   National Health Insurance Fund for Salaried Workers (Caisse Nationale d'Assurance Maladie des Travailleurs Salariés)

CNPF   Confederation of French Employers (Confédération Nationale du Patronat Français)

CSMF   Confederation of French Medical Trade Unions (Confédération des Syndicats Médicaux Français)

DDASS   Local Public Health Administration (Direction Départementale des Affaires Sanitaires et Sociales)

DRASS   Regional Public Health Administration (Direction Régionale des Affaires Sanitaires et Sociales)

FMF   Federation of French Physicians (Fédération des Médecins de France)

GDP   Gross Domestic Product

GIH   Cooperative Union of Hospitals (Groupement Interhospitalier)

INSEE   National Institute for Statistical and Economic Studies (Institut Nationale des Etudes Statistiques et Economiques)

| NHI | National Health Insurance |
| RCB | French Program Planning and Budgeting System - PPBS (Rationalisation des Choix Budgétaires) |

Québec

CLSC	Local Health and Social Service Center (Centre Local de Services Communautaires)
CRSSS	Regional Council for Health and Social Services (Conseil Régional de la Santé et des Services Sociaux)
CSS	Social Service Center (Centre de Services Sociaux)
DSC	Department of Community Health (Département de Santé Communautaire)
QHIB	Québec Health Insurance Board (Régie de l'Assurance Maladie du Québec)

England

AHA	Area Health Authority
BG	Board of Governors
BMA	British Medical Association
CMC	Community Health Council
DHSS	Department of Health and Social Security
DMT	District Management Team
FPC	Family Practice Committee
GP	General Practitioner
HMC	Hospital management committee
JCC	Joint Consultative Committee
MPC	Medical Practices Committee

NHS	National Health Service
PESC	Public Expenditure Survey Committee
RAWP	Resource Allocation Working Party
RHA	Regional Health Authority
RHB	Regional Hospital Board

United States

CON	Certificate of Need
CHP	Comprehensive Health Planning
DHHS	Department of Health and Human Services
DRG	Diagnosis Related Group
HCFA	Health Care Financing Administration
HMO	Health Maintenance Organization
HRA	Health Resources Administration
HSA	Health Systems Agency
NHC	Neighborhood Health Center
PPO	Preferred Provider Organization
PSRO	Professional Standards Review Organization
SHCC	State Health Coordinating Council
SHPDA	State Health Planning and Development Agency

NOTES

1. THE NATURE OF HEALTH PLANNING

1. The notion of a "medical industrial complex" was originally used by Barbara and John Ehrenreich in a book they prepared for Health-Pac: *The American Health Empire: Power, Profits and Politics* (New York: Random House, Vintage Edition, 1970), chap. VII. The notion was adopted—albeit with some differences in interpretation—by the editor of the *New England Journal of Medicine*. See A. Relman, "The New Medical-Industrial Complex," *New England Journal of Medicine*, 303, 17 (1980), 963–970.

2. S. Cohen and C. Goldfinger, "From Real Crisis to Permacrisis in French Social Security," in R. Alford, C. Crouch, L. Lindberg, and C. Offe, eds., *Stress and Contradiction in Modern Capitalism* (Lexington, Mass.: D. C. Heath, 1975).

3. L. Hirshhorn, "The Theory of Social Services in Disaccumulationist Capitalism," *International Journal of Health Services*, 9, 2 (1979), 295–311; and "The Political Economy of Social Service Rationalization: A Developmental View," *Contemporary Crisis* 2 (1978), 63–81.

4. J. Weinstein, *The Corporate Ideal in the Liberal State: 1900–1918* (Boston: Beacon Press, 1968).

5. K. Mannheim, *Man and Society in an Age of Reconstruction* (New York: Harcourt, Brace & World, Inc., 1940).

6. H. Blum, *Planning for Health*. 2d ed. (New York: Human Sciences Press, 1981).

7. L. Nizard, "Planning as the Regulatory Reproduction of the Status Quo," in J. Hayward and M. Watson, eds., *Planning, Politics and Public Policy: The British, French, and Italian Experience* (Cambridge: Cambridge University Press, 1965). Also see L. Tannen, "Health Planning as a Regulatory Strategy: A Discussion of Current History and Current Uses," *International Journal of Health Services* (Winter 1979); and Louanne Kennedy, "Health Planning in An Age of Austerity," in R. Straetz, M. Lieberman and A. Sardell, *Critical Issues in Health Policy* (Lexington, Mass.: D. C. Heath, 1981).

8. E. Krause, "Health Planning as a Managerial Ideology," *International Journal of Health Services* 3, 3 (1973).

9. R. Alford, *Health Care Politics* (Chicago: University of Chicago Press, 1975), p. 176.

10. A. Wildavsky, "If Planning is Everything, Maybe It's Nothing," *Policy Sciences* 4 (1973), 127—153.

11. S. Cohen, "From Causation to Decision: Planning as Politics," *American Economic Review* (May 1970), pp. 180—185.

12. M. Webber, "The Prospects for Policies Planning," in L. Duhl, ed., *The Urban Condition* (New York: Basic Books, 1963), pp. 319—330.

13. J. Forester, "Planning in the Face of Power," *Journal of the American Planning Association* 48, 1 (1982), 67—80; and "Questioning and Organizing Attention: Toward a Critical Theory of Planning and Administrative Practice," *Administration and Society*, 13, 2 (1981), 161—205.

14. A. Wildavsky, "Can Health Be Planned?" Michael Davis lecture, Center for Health Administration, Graduate School of Business, University of Chicago, 1976.

15. J. Wilson, "An Overview of Theories of Planned Change," in R. Morris, ed., *Centrally Planned Change* (New York: National Association of Social Workers, 1964), p. 29.

16. Ibid., p. 21.

17. Existing theory on the nature of planning is not precisely formulated. It is difficult, therefore, to test hypotheses without sacrificing substantive issues for methodological rigor. For this reason, this study adopts a comparative case study approach. Case studies, of course, cannot be used to prove general propositions; their traditional claim is to emphasize the potential for providing "in-depth" analysis. In contrast to cross-national, aggregate statistical analysis, case studies provide a context in which to combine historical, political, economic, and social perspectives. Moreover, they provide a way to tell the story of how health planning emerged and now operates in France, Québec, and England.

2. HEALTH PLANNING AND THE STATE

1. A. Shonfield, *Modern Capitalism: The Changing Balance of Public and Private Power* (Cambridge: Cambridge University Press, 1965).

2. P. Massé, *Le Plan ou l'Anti-Hasard* (Paris: Gallimard, 1965).

3. R. Heilbroner, *Business Civilization in Decline* (New York: Norton, 1976); J. Galbraith, *Economics and the Public Purpose* (Boston: Houghton Mifflin Co., 1973). Also see A. Shonfield, *The Use of Public Power* (New York: Oxford University Press, 1982).

4. D. Bell, *The Coming of Post-Industrial Society: A Venture in Social Forecasting* (New York: Basic Books, 1973). For a provocative discussion of the problems raised by explosive service sector growth, see W. Baumol, "The Macroeconomics of Unbalanced Growth: Anatomy of the Urban

Crisis," *American Economic Review* 57 (June 1967), 415—426; and L. Hirshhorn, "Toward a Political Economy of the Service Society" (Berkeley: University of California, Institute of Urban and Regional Development, Working Paper, No. 229), 1974.

5. United States Department of Commerce, Bureau of the Census, *Statistical Abstract of the United States, 1974* (Washington, D.C.: Government Printing Office, 1974), table 604.

6. I have discussed this point in some detail in my paper on "Health Insurance and Alcohol Treatment Services: A Strategy for Change or a Buttress for the Status Quo?" Paper presented at the American Public Health Association, Montreal, 1982.

7. Medical care is only one determinant of health; other more important determinants include genetic, behavioral, environmental, as well as social and economic factors (see Appendix 1, fig. 15). Such is the conventional wisdom in the field of public health. See e.g., R. Dubos, *Man Adapting* (New Haven: Yale University Press, 1965) and T. McKeown, *Medicine in Modern Society* (London: Allen & Unwin, 1965). More specifically, on the limits of modern medicine, see A. Cochrane, *Effectiveness and Efficiency, Random Reflections on Health Services* (London: Oxford University Press for the Nuffield Provincial Hospitals Trust, 1972) and J. Powles, "On the Limitations of Modern Medicine," *Science, Medicine and Man* 1 (1973), 1—30.

8. M. Lerner and R. Stutz, "Have We Narrowed the Gaps Between the Poor and the Non-Poor?" *Medical Care* 15, 8 (1977).

9. J. Geisel, "Cost of Employee Benefits Soars 763% Over 30 Years," *Business Insurance*, August 17, 1981, p. 3.

10. *Public Expenditure on Health*, no. 4 (Paris: OECD Studies in Resource Allocation, July 1977), p. 28.

11. OECD, Directorate of Social Affairs, Manpower and Education, "The Evolution of Public Expenditure on Health" mimeo, March 8, 1982.

12. M. Rein, "Policy Analysis as an Interpretation of Beliefs," *Journal of the Institute of American Planners* 37, 5 (1971).

13. In addition to the empirical and heuristic aspects of science, Gerald Holton observes that there are "dimensions of fundamental presuppositions, notions, terms, methodological judgments and decisions—in short, of themata or themes—which are themselves neither directly evolved from, nor resolvable into, objective observation on the one hand, or logical, mathematical and other formal analytical ratiocination on the other hand." *Thematic Origins of Scientific Thought* (Cambridge: Harvard University Press, 1973), p. 50. I have cited Holton here but similar ideas have been expressed by others. See e.g., T. Kuhn, *The Structure of Scientific Revolutions* (Chicago: University of Chicago Press, 1970) and P. Feyerabend, *Against Method* (London: NLB, 1975). For provocative essays on the implications of such views for the growth of knowledge, see

I. Lakatos and A. Musgrave, eds., *Criticism and the Growth of Knowledge* (London: Cambridge University Press, 1970).

14. These three terms have been used by different authors in various ways. For more detail on the tradition of conservative, radical, and liberal world views, see, above all, B. Ward, *The Ideal Worlds of Economics* (New York: Basic Books, 1979). Also, see R. Alford, "Paradigms of Relations Between State and Society," in L. Lindberg et al., eds., *Stress and Contradiction in Modern Capitalism* (Lexington, Mass.: D. H. Heath, 1975) and D. Gordon, ed., *Problems in Political Economy: An Urban Perspective* (Lexington: D. C. Heath, 1971), chapters 1 and 6.

15. E. Burke, *Reflections on the Revolution in France* (Garden City, N.Y.: Doubleday & Co., 1961); J. S. Mill, "On Liberty," in M. Lerner, ed., *Essential Works of J. S. Mill* (New York: Bantam, 1961); A. Smith, *An Inquiry into the Nature and Causes of the Wealth of Nations* (New York: Modern Library, 1937).

16. M. Friedman, "The Role of Government in a Free Society," in *Capitalism and Freedom* (Chicago: University of Chicago Press, 1962), p. 23.

17. Ibid.

18. Ibid.

19. Today there is a flourishing literature in this tradition. See, e.g., J. Habermas, *Legitimation Crisis* (Boston: Beacon Press, 1973); R. Miliband, *The State in Capitalist Society* (London: Quartet Books, 1973); J. O'Connor, *The Fiscal Crisis of the State* (New York: St. Martin's Press, 1973); C. Offe, "Structural Problems of the Capitalist State," in K. von Beyme, ed., *German Political Studies* (London: Russel Sage, 1974); C. Offe, "The Theory of the Capitalist State and the Problem of Policy Formation," in L. Lindberg et al., eds., *Stress and Contradiction*; and N. Poulantzas, *Political Power and Social Classes* (London: New Left Books, 1978).

20. P. Sweezy, "The Radical Theory of the State," in D. Gordon, ed., *Problems in Political Economy: An Urban Perspective*, p. 25.

21. K. Marx and F. Engels, *The Communist Manifesto*.

22. J. Habermas, *Legitimation Crisis*.

23. J. O'Connor, *Fiscal Crisis*.

24. C. Offe, "The Theory of the Capitalist State."

25. Ibid., p. 143.

26. B. Ward, *The Liberal Economic World View* (New York: Basic Books, 1979).

27. R. Tawney, *The Radical Tradition*, cited by A. Donabedian, *Aspects of Medical Care Administration: Specifying Requirements for Health Care* (Cambridge: Harvard University Press, 1973), pp. 260, 261, 267.

28. R. Dahl and C. Lindblom, *Politics, Economics and Welfare* (New York: Harper and Brothers, 1953); J. Galbraith, *The New Industrial State* (New York: Houghton Mifflin, 1967); R. Musgrave, *The Theory of Public Finance* (New York: McGraw Hill, 1959); G. Myrdal, *Beyond the Welfare*

State (New Haven: Yale University Press, 1960); A. Shonfield, *Modern Capitalism*; R. Titmus, *Essays on the Welfare State* (Boston: Beacon Press, 1969).

29. W. Heller, "Reflections on Public Expenditure Theory," in D. Gordon, ed., *Problems in Political Economy*, p. 39.

30. R. Alford, "Paradigms of Relations Between State and Society."

31. As noted in chapter 1, planning is often defined as an administrative mechanism for replacing the market. However, this is not its only function. In some cases, for example, antitrust policy and certain government regulations, planning can serve to foster market competition. Even if planning reduces the role of economic markets, there might, nevertheless, remain significant competition in the form of political markets, e.g., when organized interests put pressure on elected representatives or when logrolling occurs in regional health planning bodies.

32. M. Lynch and S. Raphael, *Medicine and the State* (Springfield, Ill.: Charles Thomas, 1963), p. 422.

33. Cited in ibid., p. 414.

34. D. Lees, "Health Through Choice," in R. Harris, ed., *Freedom or Free-for-all* (London: Institute of Economic Affairs, 1968); M. Friedman, *Capitalism and Freedom*, chap. 9.

35. M. Friedman, *Capitalism and Freedom*, p. 158. Physicians are, in fact, liable for any injury which is the proximate cause of their negligence where negligence is established by the standard of what the ordinary physician would do under similar circumstances. In addition, physicians may be liable for subjecting patients to risk without informed consent. The widespread presence of insurance against malpractice, however, raises questions as to whether insurance actually deters negligence when the physician does not bear the full financial consequences of his negligence.

36. R. Kessel, "Price Discrimination in Medicine," *Journal of Law and Economics* 1 (October 1958).

37. M. Friedman, *Capitalism and Freedom*, pp. 158–159.

38. See, e.g., V. Navarro, "Political Power, the State, and Their Implications in Medicine," and J. Salmon, "Monopoly Capital and the Reorganization of the Health Sector," *The Review of Radical Political Economics* 9, 1 (1977).

39. See, e.g., B. and J. Ehrenreich, *The American Health Empire: Power, Profits and Politics* (New York: Random House, 1970).

40. For an economic analysis of how medical care is different from other goods and services, see K. Arrow, "Uncertainty and the Welfare Economics of Medical Care," *American Economic Review* 53, 5 (December 1963). Also, see A. Culyer, "Is Medical Care Different?" in M. Cooper and A. Culyer, eds., *Health Economics* (Middlesex, England: Penguin, 1973).

41. Cited by M. Lynch and S. Raphael, *Medicine and the State*, p. 8.

42. G. B. Shaw, *Doctor's Dilemma* (London: Constable, 1930), preface.

43. M. Lynch and S. Raphael, *Medicine and the State*, p. 9.

44. I. Illich, *Medical Nemesis: The Expropriation of Health* (London: Calder and Boyars, 1975).

45. Illich's critique of industrialism has annoyed Marxist analysts in the health field and has led the French magazine, Le Nouvel Observateur, to call Illich a "petit réactionnaire." See, e.g., V. Navarro, "The Industrialization of Fetishism or the Fetishism of Industrialization: A Critique of Ivan Illich," in V. Navarro, *Health and Medical Care in the U.S.: A Critical Analysis* (Farmingdale, N.Y.: Baywood Publishing Co., 1973).

46. I. Illich, "Two Watersheds," in *Tools for Conviviality* (New York: Pantheon, 1973), p. 6.

47. I. Illich, *Medical Nemesis*, p. 165.

48. K. Arrow, "Uncertainty and the Welfare Economics of Medical Care," *American Economic Review* 53 (1963) 941–973; A. Culyer, "The Nature of the Commodity 'Health Care' and Its Efficient Allocation," *Oxford Economic Papers* 23 (1971), 189–211.

49. A. Culyer, "The 'Market' Versus the 'State' in Medical Care," in G. McLachlan, ed., *Problems and Progress in Medical Care* (London: Oxford University Press, 1972), p. 6. Also, see A. Culyer, "The NHS and the Market: Images and Realities," in G. McLachlan and A. Maynard, eds., *The Public/Private Mix for Health* (London: The Nuffield Provincial Hospitals Trust, 1982).

50. M. Weber, *The Theory of Social and Economic Organization*, trans. A. Henderson (New York: Free Press, 1968).

51. On the notion of rights, see R. Dworkin, *Taking Rights Seriously* (Cambridge: Harvard University Press, 1977). On the notion of justice, see J. Rawls, *A Theory of Justice* (Cambridge: Harvard University Press, 1971).

52. I am grateful to the Reverend Paul Lehmann for bringing this formulation to my attention.

3. HEALTH PLANNING AND IMPLEMENTATION

1. See, e.g., H. Blum, *Planning for Health*, 2d ed. (New York: Human Sciences Press, 1981); H. Hyman, *Health Planning: A Systematic Approach* (Germantown, Md.: Aspen Systems Corporation, 1975); and A. Donabedian, *Aspects of Medical Care Administration: Specifying Requirements for Health Care* (Cambridge: Harvard University Press, 1973). For a discussion focused more on the concept of need, also see K. Boulding, "The Concept of Need for Health Services," *Milbank Memorial Fund Quarterly* 2 (1966); J. Bradshaw, "A Taxonomy of Social Need," in G. McLachlan, ed., *Problems and Progress in Medical Care* (London: Oxford University

Press, 1972); A. Culyer, *Need and the National Health Service: Economics and Social Choice* (London: Martin Robertson, 1976).

2. Some observers have attempted to explain such variation based on a collaborative cross-national study of the determinants of health care utilization (R. Kohn and K. White, eds., *Health Care: An International Study* [London: Oxford University Press, 1976]). Others merely interpret such variation as evidence of the cultural specificity of medical care organization (J. de Kervasdoué, "Les politiques de santé sont-elles adaptées à la pratique médicale," *Sociologie du Travail*, 3 [1979]). Whether such variation is attributable to differences in perceived morbidity is an interesting question for a doctoral dissertation. My point here is merely to establish that there are important differences in medical care organization.

3. Relying heavily on unpublished writings of J. Dyckman, M. Meyerson, H. Gans, and N. Glazer, A. Blackman has written a useful summary of the virtues and defects of standards in health planning: "The Meaning and Use of Standards," in H. Blum and Associates, *Health Planning 1969* (San Francisco: APHA, Western Regional Office), chap. 4.

4. N. Glazer, *Health Planning, Science, Power and Politics* (Berkeley: University of California, Institute of Urban and Regional Development, Monograph No. 16, Jan. 1970), p. 2.

5. In a general analysis of the problem of planning and implementation in the health sector, Altenstetter and Björkman note, "Typically, planning officials do not plan for implementation. Rather, they wax eloquent on goals and preferred end-states, and assume that the means of implementation will be forthcoming." C. Altenstetter and J. Björkman, "Planning and Implementation: A Comparative Perspective on Health Policy" (Berlin: International Institute of Management, 1978), p. 34.

6. E. Bardach, *The Implementation Game: What Happens after a Bill Becomes a Law* (Cambridge: MIT Press, 1977), chap. 2.

7. The first formulation is the subtitle of E. Bardach's book, ibid. The second formulation is by M. Rein and F. Rabinovitz, "Implementation: A Theoretical Perspective" (Cambridge: Joint Center for Urban Studies, Working Paper No. 43, March 1977), p. 1.

8. J. Pressman and A. Wildavsky, *Implementation* (Berkeley, Los Angeles, London: University of California Press, 1973), p. 107.

9. E. Bardach, *Implementation Game*, p. 3.

10. Ibid., p. 283.

11. H. Heclo, "Frontiers of Social Policy in Europe and America," *Policy Sciences* 6 (1975), 413–414.

12. For a clear presentation of the distinction between "decision making" and "agenda setting," see P. Bachrach and M. Baratz, "Decisions and Nondecisions: An Analytical Framework," *American Political Science Review* 56 (1962), 642–651.

13. Parts of the section on medical care system behavior have been inspired by W. McClure, "The Medical Care System Under National Health Insurance: Four Models," in K. Friedman and S. Rakoff, *Toward A National Health Policy* (Lexington, Mass.: D. C. Heath, 1977).

14. J. Ellul, *Le système technicien* (Paris: Calmann Lévy, 1977), my translation.

15. A. Wildavsky, "Doing Better and Feeling Worse: The Political Pathology of Health Policy," *Daedalus* (Winter 1977).

16. A. Dobson et al., "PSROs: Their Current Status and Their Impact to Date," *Inquiry* 15, 2 (1978), 113—128.

17. S. Schroeder and J. Showstack, "Financial Incentives to Perform Medical Procedures and Laboratory Tests: Illustrative Models of Office Practice," *Medical Care* 16 (1978), 289—298; J. Showstack et al., "Fee-for-Service Physician Payment: Analysis of Current Methods and Their Development," *Inquiry* 16 (1979), 230—246.

18. A. Parker, "Dimensions of Primary Care," in S. Andreopoulos, ed., *Primary Care: Where Medicine Fails* (New York: John Wiley and Sons, 1974), p. 61.

19. For two opposing views on this point, see V. Navarro, "National Health Insurance and the Strategy for Change," *Milbank Mem. Fund Q.* 51, 2 (1973), 223—251; and M. Roemer, "Social Insurance as a Leverage for Changing Health Care Systems: International Experience," *Bull. of the N. Y. Acad. of Med.* 48, 1 (1972), 93—107.

20. This section draws on an analysis by U. Reinhardt, "Alternative Methods of Reimbursing Non-institutional Providers of Health Services," in *Controls on Health Care*, Papers of the Conference on Regulation in the Health Industry, January 9, 1974 (Washington, D.C.: National Academy of Sciences, 1975).

21. M. Roemer and W. Shonick, "HMO Performance: The Recent Evidence," *Milbank Mem. Fund Q.* 51 (1973), 271—317. For a more comprehensive view, see H. Luft, *Health-Maintenance Organizations: Dimensions of Performance* (New York: John Wiley & Sons, 1981).

22. J. Bunker, "A Comparison of Operations and Surgeons in the United States and in England and Wales." *New England Journal of Medicine*, 282, 3 (1970), pp. 135—144.

23. M. Blumberg, "Rational Provider Prices: An Incentive for Improved Health Delivery," in G. Chacko, ed., *Health Handbook* (Amsterdam: North Holland, 1979); G. Monsma, "Marginal Revenue and the Demand for Physicians' Services," in H. Klarman, ed., *Empirical Studies in Health Economics* (Baltimore: Johns Hopkins Press, 1970). For a literature review on the impact of reimbursement incentives on physician behavior, see H. Luft, "Economic Incentives and Clinical Decisions," in B. Gray, ed., *The New Health Care for Profit* (Washington, D.C.: National Academy Press, 1983).

24. W. Dowling, "Prospective Reimbursement of Hospitals," *Inquiry*

11 (1974), 163–180; J. Lave, L. Lave, and L. Silverman, "A Proposal for Incentive Reimbursement for Hospitals," *Medical Care* 11, 79 (1973); C. McCarthy, "Incentive Reimbursement as an Impetus to Cost Containment," *Inquiry* 11 (1975); M. Pauly, "Efficiency, Incentives, and Reimbursement for Health Care," *Inquiry* 7, 14 (1970).

25. The results of these experiments are reported by T. Galblum, *Research in Health Care Financing* (Washington, D.C.: U.S. DHEW Publication No. [SSA] 77-1190, 1977).

26. See, e.g., U. Reinhardt, *Physician Productivity and the Demand for Health Manpower* (Cambridge, Mass.: Ballinger, 1975), chap. 1; F. Golladay and M. Manser, "Studies of the Determination of the Spatial Distribution of Physicians," Health Economics Research Paper no. 4 (Madison: University of Wisconsin, 1970); and G. Rimlinger and H. Steele, "An Economic Interpretation of the Spatial Distribution of Physicians in the U. S.," *Southern Economic Journal* 30 (1963).

27. I. Burney et al., "Medicare and Medicaid Physician Payment Incentives," *Health Care Financing Review* (Summer 1979), p. 68.

28. This table was inspired by Eugene Bardach in the course of a discussion with C. Davies, J. de Kervasdoué, R. Klein, T. Marmor, and J. C. Stephan, on the occasion of the "Conference on Health and Disease in Industrialized Nations in 1995," Megève, France, January 5–9, 1979.

29. See, e.g., C. Havighurst, ed., *Regulating Health Facilities Construction. (Proceedings of a Conference on Health Planning, Certificate of Need, and Market Entry)* (Washington, D.C.: American Enterprise Institute for Public Policy Research, 1974); and *Controls on Health Care.*

30. K. Davis, "Health and the Great Society: Successes of the Past Decade and the Road Ahead," in D. Warner, ed., *Toward A New Human Rights: The Social Policies of the Kennedy and Johnson Administrations* (Austin: University of Texas Press, 1977).

31. K. Bauer, *Cost Containment Under P.L. 93-641: Strengthening the Partnership Between Health Planning and Regulation. Final Report* (Cambridge: Harvard University Center for Community Health and Medical Care, January 1978), p. 29.

32. W. Glaser, *Paying the Doctor: Systems of Remuneration and Their Effects* (Baltimore: Johns Hopkins Press, 1970).

33. P. Feldstein, "An Analysis of Reimbursement Plans," in *Reimbursement Incentives for Hospital and Medical Care* (Washington, D.C.: Social Security Administration, Research Report 26, 1968).

4. PROFILES OF HEALTH SYSTEMS

1. For a succinct review of the role of the federal government in the American health system, see P. Lee, "Role of the Federal Government in

Health and Medical Affairs," *New England Journal of Medicine*, 279 (1968), 1139−1147.

2. Collective financing refers to all financing coming from third-party payers: Social Security, private health insurance, and/or government. In France, national health insurance covers most of the costs, whereas in the United States they are covered by private health insurance and government programs.

3. J. Hayward, "Solidarity: The Social History of an Idea in Nineteenth Century France," *International Journal of Social History* IV, 2 (1959), 261−284.

4. I have elaborated on this point in my "The Marriage of National Health Insurance and *La Médecine Libérale* in France: A Costly Union," *Milbank Mem. Fund Q.* 51, 1 (1981).

5. T. Marmor, A. Bridges, and W. Hoffman, "Comparative Politics and Health Policies," in D. Ashford, ed., *Comparing Public Policies* (Beverly Hills: Sage Publications, 1977), p. 65.

6. M. Renaud, "Political Economy of Québec State Interventions in Health: Reform or Revolution" (Dissertation proposal, University of Wisconsin, Madison, 1975), p. 3.

7. M. Cooper, "Economics of Need: The Experience of the British Health Service," in M. Perlman, ed., *The Economics of Health and Medical Care* (New York: John Wiley and Sons, 1974), p. 90.

8. Consultative Council on Medical and Allied Services, *Interim Report on the Future Position of Medical and Allied Services* (London: Her Majesty's Stationery Office, 1920).

9. Royal Commission on National Health Insurance, *Report* (London: Her Majesty's Stationery Office, Command No. 2596, 1926).

10. British Medical Association, *A General Medical Service for the Nation* (London: BMA, 1938).

11. W. Beveridge, *Report on Social Insurance and Allied Services* (London: Her Majesty's Stationery Office); cited in S. Harris, "The British Health Experiment: The First Two Years of the National Health Service," *American Economic Review* 41, 2 (May 1951), 652.

12. V. Navarro, *Class Struggle, The State and Medicine: An Historical and Contemporary Analysis of the Medical Sector in Great Britain* (New York: Prodist, 1978), chap. 4.

13. O. Anderson, *Health Care: Can There be Equity? The United States, Sweden, and England* (New York: John Wiley and Sons, 1972), p. 93.

14. V. Navarro, *Class Struggle*, p. 47.

15. The literal translation of CNAMTS is the National Sickness Insurance Fund of Salaried Workers. Since the more customary American term for sickness insurance is health insurance, I have taken the liberty of referring to French NHI.

16. Ministry of Health, *Recensement des établissements d'hospitalisation*

privée-activité et personnel, Division d'Etudes et du Plan, 1973, and *Bulletin de Statistiques* 6, b (1973).

17. H. Blum, *Expanding Health Care Horizons: From a General Systems Concept of Health to a National Health Policy* (Oakland: Third Party Associates, Inc., 1976), chap. 7.

18. R. Klein, "Ideology, Class and the National Health Service," *Journal of Health Politics, Policy and Law*, 4, 3 (1979). The data are drawn from this article.

19. M. Cooper, *Rationing Health Care* (New York: John Wiley and Sons, 1975).

20. For a thorough review of this form of physician remuneration, see J. Showstack, et al., "Fee-for-Service Physician Payment: Analysis of Current Methods and Their Development," *Inquiry* 16, 3 (1979), 230–246.

21. Review Body on Doctors' and Dentists' Remuneration, *Fourth Report* (London: Her Majesty's Stationary Office, 1974), p. 41; cited in R. Klein, "Ideology, Class."

22. C. Davies, "Hospital Centered Health Care: Policies and Politics in the NHS," in P. Atkinson, et al., eds., *Prospects for the National Health* (London: Croom Helm, 1979).

23. C. Davies, "The Dynamic of Hospital Centered Health Care: Data and Arguments from the British Case," paper for presentation to the European Group on Organization Studies, Health Organizations Group Conference on Different Conceptions of Health Care Systems: Alternatives to a Hospital Centered Orientation (Augsburg, November 1977).

24. H. Eckstein, *The English Health Service: Its Origins, Structure and Achievement* (Cambridge: Harvard University Press, 1959).

25. P. Fox, "Managing Health Resources: English Style," in G. McLachlan, ed., *By Guess or By What? Information Without Design in the NHS* (Oxford: Nuffield Provincial Hospitals Trust, 1978).

26. W. Glaser, *Health Insurance Bargaining: Foreign Lessons for Americans* (New York: John Wiley and Sons, Inc., 1978), chap. 9.

27. Cited by V. Navarro, *Class Struggle, the State and Medicine* (New York: Prodist, 1978), p. 41.

5. HEALTH PLANNING UNDER NATIONAL HEALTH INSURANCE: FRANCE

1. P. Samuelson, *Economics* 10th ed. (New York: McGraw Hill, 1976), p. 873.

2. P. Massé, "The Guiding Ideas Behind French Planning," *French Affairs* (New York: French Consulate, 1962).

3. S. Cohen, *Modern Capitalist Planning: The French Model* (Cambridge:

Harvard University Press, 1969).

4. For elaboration on French national economic planning, see the chapters in J. Hayward and M. Watson, eds., *Planning, Politics and Public Policy: The British, French, and Italian Experience* (Cambridge: Cambridge University Press, 1965); and A. Shonfield, *Modern Capitalism: The Changing Balance of Public and Private Power* (New York: Oxford University Press, 1965). Also, see L. Nizard, ed., *Planification et société* (Grenoble: Presses Universitaires de Grenoble, 1974).

5. The figure is cited by C. Altenstetter, "Hospital Planning in France and the Federal Republic of Germany," *Journal of Health Politics Policy and Law* 5, 2 (1980), 314. On the history of French health insurance, see R. Bridgman, "Medical Care Under Social Security in France," *International Journal of Health Services*, 4 (1971), 331−341.

6. P. Cibrie, *Syndicalisme médical* (Paris: Confédération des Syndicats Médicaux Français, 1954), p. 68.

7. For more detail on these issues, see W. Glaser, *Paying the Doctor: Systems of Remuneration and their Effects* (Baltimore: Johns Hopkins Press, 1970), pp. 124−134; and W. Glaser, *Health Insurance Bargaining* (New York: Gardner Press, Inc., 1978), pp. 39−55.

8. Originally written by the CSMF in 1930, the fee schedule (nomenclature) classifies medical procedures by so-called key letters: C, Cs, and $Cpsy$ signify consultations with general practitioners, specialists, and psychiatrists, respectively; V, Vs, and $Vpsy$ signify home visits by general practitioners, specialists, and psychiatrists; B signifies laboratory tests; Z signifies all radiological procedures; and K signifies surgical and specialty procedures. The Bs, Zs, and Ks are always followed by a coefficient that is supposed to reflect their relative value on an elaborate scale of medical procedures. For example, an appendectomy or simple hernia operation is coded as K-50, whereas the surgical removal of an ingrown toenail is coded as K-10. Physician fees are equal to the coefficient times the value of the key letters, which serve as the explicit object of bargaining during the national fee negotiation. The most recent version of the nomenclature is published in *La Revue du Praticien* 29, 17 (March 1979), 1−154. As of February 1979, the C, Cs, and $Cpsy$ were equal to 40, 60, and 92 francs; the V, Vs, and $Vpsy$ were equal to 53, 71, and 103 francs; the K was equal to 8.30 francs; and the Z, to 5.20 francs.

9. For an incisive analysis of the evolving relationships between physicians' trade unions and the state, see J. C. Stephan, *Economie et pouvoir médical* (Paris: Economica, 1978).

10. H. Hatzfeld, *Le grand tournant de la médicine libérale* (Paris: Editions Ouvrières, 1963), p. 293.

11. F. Steudler, "L'évolution de la profession médicale: essai d'analyse sociologique," *Cahiers de Sociologie et de Démographie Médicales*, 2 (April−June 1973).

12. J. C. Stephan, *Economie et pouvoir médical*.

13. H. Hatzfeld, *Le grand tournant.*

14. H. Jamous, *Sociologie de la décision: la réforme des études médicales et des structures hospitalières* (Paris: Centre National de la Recherche Scientifique [CNRS], 1969).

15. Cited by H. Hatzfeld, *Le grand tournant*, p. 297; translation: "Do you understand that it is impossible for you to remain entirely individualistic in a society that is moving toward collective forms of organization?"

16. Under the present socialist government, this privilege has been revoked.

17. J. de Kervasdoué, "La politique de l'Etat en matière d'hospitalisation privée. 1962—1978. analyse des conséquences de mesures contradictoires," *Annales Economiques de Clermont-Ferrand.* 16 (1979), 25—56.

18. *Le Monde*, January 10, 1979, article by N. Beau.

19. From 1974—1981 the number of beds in the public sector increased at a rate of 1.9 percent whereas in the private sector they increased at a rate of 9 percent. See J. de Kervasdoué, *Les politiques de santé et l'evolution des dépenses*, Document no. 16, Commission on Labor (Paris: CGP, November 25, 1982), mimeo.

20. E. Lévy et al., *Hospitalisation publique, hospitalisation privée* (Paris: Centre National de Recherche Scientifique, no. 22, 1977).

21. J. de Kervasdoué, "La politique de l'Etat en matière d'hospitalisation privée."

22. F. Steudler, *L'hôpital en observation* (Paris: Armand Colin, 1974).

23. See articles in *Le Monde* (June 12 and August 25, 1976).

24. For arguments in support of the private sector, see, e.g., the publications of the Fédération Intersyndicale des Etablissements d'Hospitalisation Privée (FIEHP). For a defense of the public sector, see *Fédération Hospitalière de France* (FHF), *L'hôpital public coûte-t-il plus cher que les cliniques privées?* (Paris: FHF, 1976.)

25. M. Castaing, "L'hôpital, ce malade chronique," *Le Monde* (Feb. 21, 1975).

26. In 1973, the image of l'Assistance Publique (AP) in Paris sank so low that the central administration ran spots on television, in movie theaters, and in the daily press, the purpose of which was to *sensibiliser l'opinion publique.* On April 8, *l'opération découvrez vos hôpitaux* was launched, bringing 70,000 to 80,000 Parisians to twenty-eight of AP's thirty-seven hospitals (*Rapport annuel*, Paris: AP 1973).

27. *Tableaux, santé et sécurité sociale* (Paris: Documentation Française, 1975), p. 261.

28. "Situation des hôpitaux publics," memorandum of the Fédération Hospitalière Française to the Ministry of Health and Social Security, in *Revue Hospitalière de France* (1973), p. 665.

29. E. Errahmani, *Contribution à la carte hospitalière de la région parisienne* (Paris: Cahiers de l'Institut d'Aménagement et d'Urbanisme de la Région Parisienne, 1972), vol. 29.

30. E. Errahmani, "Note sur la concentration géographique de l'équipement hospitalier de la région parisienne" (Paris: Observatoire Régional de la Santé, March 5, 1975).

31. *Rapport géneral de la commission des prestations sociales.* Fifth National Economic Plan (Paris: Documentaion Française, 1966).

32. "Pour une réforme hospitalière, rapport presenté par M. Roger Grégoire," in *Pour une politique de la santé. rapports présentés à Robert Boulin* (Paris: Documentation Française, 1970).

33. *Réflexions sur l'avenir de système de santé. rapport du groupe de travail sur la prospective de la santé.* (Paris: Documentation Française, 1969).

34. M. Chapalain, "La rationalisation des choix budgétaires au ministère de la santé," *Cahiers de Sociologie et de Démographie Médicale,* 2 (April – June 1975).

35. M. Chapalain, "Perinatality: French Cost-Benefit Studies and Decisions on Handicap and Prevention," *Ciba Foundation Symposium,* 59 (1978).

36. For an insightful essay on RCB and on the state of social planning in France, see B. Jobert, "Aspects of Social Planning in France," in J. Hayward and O. Narkiewicz, eds., *Planning in Europe* (London: Croom Helm, 1978).

37. F. Villey, *La réforme hospitalière. notes et études documentaires* (Paris: Documentation Française, 1977).

38. C. Brumter, *La planification sanitaire* (Strasbourg: Université des Sciences Juridiques, Politiques, Sociales et de Technologie, Faculté de Droit et de Sciences Politiques, February 1979).

39. "Un décrêt permet aux cliniques privées 'à but non lucratif' de participer au service hospitalier public," *Le Monde* (May 27, 1976).

40. *Comptes nationaux de la santé* (Paris: Centre de Recherche pour l'Etude et l'Observation des Conditions de Vie (CREDOC), 1982).

41. Figures 4–6 are based on estimates from the French National Health Accounts compiled by CREDOC. Final medical care consumption (CMF) represents the greater part of aggregate health expenditures including categorical programs such as maternal and child health, school and university programs, the health service for the military, biomedical research, administrative costs, and capital formation. In figures 5 and 6, CMF is deflated by the 1970 general price inflation index used by the Institut National des Etudes Statistiques et Economiques (INSEE). In figure 6, the growth of the CNAMTS' expenditures is always higher than those of the CMF because they are more sensitive to the growth in hospital expenditures and because health insurance coverage has increased over the past two decades.

In looking over the growth rates of average annual health care costs, it is worthwhile examining the peaks and slumps in figures 4–6 for they reflect the broader forces which appear to affect the growth of health care costs: hospital investment policies, macroeconomic stabilization policy (particularly wage levels since 70 percent of hospital costs are attributed to personnel), and political events.

The peak in 1960 probably corresponds to the initial stability of the Fifth Republic and to the individual contracts signed with physicians, which assured them of reimbursement in return for acceptance of nationally set fees. The slump in 1964 is probably a reflection of former Finance Minister Giscard d'Estaing's deflationary stabilization program of 1963. The slump of 1968 appears to reflect what the French refer to as the "Events of May" as well as the earlier Social Security Reform of 1967, which tightened control over the local and regional health insurance funds. And the peak in 1969 reflects the wage increases negotiated at Grenelle following the general strike.

Although controls on hospital investment were in operation during the early seventies, their effects on growth rates in health care consumption could not possibly be detected before the late seventies for it takes 6 to 8 years, on average, to put a hospital into service from the date of initial authorization to proceed. Since the sixties and early seventies correspond to France's expansion phase in the health sector, and since wages of hospital workers increased along with hospital expansion and modernization plans, it is not surprising to note high growth rates between 1974 and 1976. As for the slump of 1973 it probably reflects the energy crisis and economic recession.

42. E. Lévy, M. Bungener, G. Duménil, and F. Fagnani, *La croissance des dépenses de santé* (Paris: Economica, 1982).

43. A recent projection by INSEE indicates that even assuming relatively high growth rates (3 percent), in 1986 the deficit for all social expenditures (health insurance, pensions, and family allowances combined) will exceed 66 billion francs and perhaps even reach 120 billion. M. Féroldi, E. Raoul, and H. Sterdyniak, "Sécurite sociale et evolution macro-économique," *Economie et Statistique* (April 1982).

44. C. Rollet, "Pourquoi modifier l'assiette des cotisations sociales?" *Droit Social* (September/October 1978).

45. A. Eugeby, "Faut-il fiscaliser la sécurité sociale?" *Droit Social*, 5 (1978).

46. Decree No. 180–188, January 8, 1980. *Journal Officiel*, 8-1, p. 65.

47. G. de Pouvourville, "La nomenclature des actes professionels, un outil pour une politique de santé?" *Revue Française des Affaires Sociales* (1981).

48. The mechanics of hospital reimbursement in France are clearly summarized by W. Glaser, *Paying the Hospital in France* (New York: Center for the Social Sciences, Columbia University, 1980).

49. These regulatory mechanisms are discussed in more detail by R. Launois and D. LeTouzé, "Analyse économique des mesures prises en

France afin de maîtriser la croissance des dépenses sanitaires," in D. Truchet, ed., *Etudes de droit et d'économie de la santé* (Paris: Economica, 1981).

50. Ibid.

51. G. Moreau, "La planification dans le domaine de la santé: les hommes et les équipements," *Revue Française des Affaires Sociales*, Numéro Spécial, no. 4, October–December 1980.

52. The two circulars date from August 1, 1977 *Bulletin Officiel de Santé Publique*—BOSP—77–34, no. 13315, and from March 3, 1978 (circular no. 536, BOSP, 78-14, no. 14658). Law no. 79-1140.

53. Ministry of Health, *Santé et sécurité sociale. tableaux* (Paris, 1972), p. 474.

54. Ministry of Health, *Annuaire des statistiques sanitaires et sociales* (Paris, 1979).

For a comprehensive guide to the French Social Security System, see, J. J. Dupéyroux, *Droit à la sécurité sociale*, 8th ed. (Paris, 1979). For a more critical appraisal of the system, see J. P. Dumont, *La sécurité sociale toujours en chantier* (Paris: Les Editions Ouvrières, 1982). Also see S. Cohen and C. Goldfinger, "From Real Crisis to Permacrisis in French Social Security," in R. Alford, C. Crouch, L. Lindberg, and C. Offe, eds., *Stress and Contradiction in Modern Capitalism* (Lexington, Mass.: D. C. Heath, 1975).

55. Finance Report. Sixth National Economic Plan (Paris: Documentation Française, 1971).

56. *Le Monde* October 15, 1976.

57. H. Galant, *Histoire politique de la sécurité sociale française* (Paris: Armand Colin, 1955).

58. This proposition is discussed at greater length in my "The Marriage of National Health Insurance and *La Médecine Libérale* in France: A Costly Union," in J. McKinlay, ed., *Politics and Health Care* (Cambridge: MIT Press, 1981).

59. R. F. Bridgman, "Hospital Regionalization in Europe: Achievements and Obstacles," in C. Altenstetter, ed., *Changing National-Subnational Relations in Health* (Washington, D.C.: Fogarty International Center, 1976).

60. *Réflexions sur l'avenir du système de santé* (Paris: Documentation Française, 1969).

61. P. Gallois and A. Taïb, eds., *De l'organisation du système de soins* (Paris: Documentation Française, 1981).

6. HEALTH PLANNING AMID INSTITUTIONAL RENOVATION: QUÉBEC

1. M. Lalonde, *A New Perspective on the Health of Canadians* (Ottawa: Government of Canada, April 1974). Also see J. Bachynsky and J. Mc-

Whinnie, "A Case Study of Canadian Planning at the Federal Level," in *Health Planning Methods: Case Studies from the 1978 International Workshop* (Washington, D.C.: DHHS, 1980, HRP-0250201, part 1); and J. Evans, "Planning and Evolution in Canadian Health Policy and Programs," in K. White and M. Henderson, eds., *Epidemiology as a Fundamental Science* (New York: Oxford University Press, 1976).

2. M. Lalonde, *A New Perspective.*

3. This point of view is shared by other observers of Canadian health policy, e.g., J. Needleman, "The Management of Medical Technology in Canada," in *The Implications of Cost-Effectiveness Analysis of Medical Technology* (Washington, D.C.: Congress of the U.S., Office of Technology Assessment, October 1980). This lies behind the reason I have chosen to focus on the case of Québec rather than on Canadian health policy as a whole, which is a good subject for another comparative study. Since Canada has a federal system of government and since health is largely a provincial responsibility, as it is between states in the United States, there is more health policy variation in Canada than in France's system of unitary government and centralized administration.

4. Figures are from M. Renaud, "Québec's New Middle Class in Search of Social Hegemony: Causes and Political Consequences," *International Review of Community Development* (1978), pp. 39–40.

5. J. Alix, "Social Change in the Health Institutions from 1960 to 1977," paper prepared for the seminar on "Social Change in Contemporary Québec," for the Department of Sociology, University of Toronto (January 1973).

6. M. Renaud, "Réforme ou illusion? une analyse des interventions de l'Etat québecois dans le domaine de la santé," in *Sociologie et Société* 9, 1 (Les Presses de l'Université de Montréal, 1977). Reprinted in D. Coburn et al., eds., *Health and Canadian Society: Sociological Perspectives* (Pickering, Ontario: Fitzhenry & Whiteside Ltd., 1979).

7. Report of the Commission of Inquiry on Health and Social Welfare (Québec: Government of Québec, 1967), Vol. I.

8. Ibid., Vol. II: *Les médecins internes et résidents* (1967) (French); Vol. III: *Development* (1971) (French and English); Vol. IV: *Health* (1970) (French and English); Vol. VI: *Les services sociaux* (1972) (French); Vol. VII: *Les professions et la santé* (1970) (French).

9. S. Lee, *Québec's Health System: A Decade of Change, 1967–1977,* Monograph No. 4 (Montreal: The Institute of Public Administration of Canada, November, 1978), p. 15.

10. The Ministry of Social Affairs has gone through several reorganizations since 1973.

11. For a thorough analysis of the new ministry's management information system, see K. Dumbaugh, *Hospital Information Systems in the Province of Québec* (Cambridge: Harvard University Center for Community Health and Medical Care, 1975).

12. Bill 65, paragraph 3, section 4.

13. For a provocative assessment of the quality of medical care in CLSCs, see M. Renaud et al., "Practice Settings and Prescribing Profiles: the Simulation of Tension Headaches to General Practitioners Working in Different Practice Settings in the Montreal Area," *American Journal of Public Health* 70, 10 (October 1980), 1068–1073.

14. This comment was made at a conference organized by Dr. Sidney Lee in 1976. Cited by S. Lee, *Quebec's Health System*, p. 41. See chap. 6 for a full report on the conference. Also, see G. Blain, ed., *La réforme des affaires sociales au québec: instruments et contraintes* (Montréal: Les Editions Administration et Santé, 1980). This book summarizes another more recent conference that evaluates Québec's health care reforms.

15. M. Taylor, *Health Insurance and Canadian Public Policy: The Seven Decisions that Created the Canadian Health Insurance System*, The Institute of Public Administration of Canada (Montreal: McGill-Queen's University Press, 1978), chap. 7.

16. *Eléments pour une politique de décentralisation administrative* (Québec: Ministère des Affaires Sociales, March 20, 1980), p. 19.

17. In summarizing Québec's experience with global budgeting, I have benefited from W. Glaser's monograph, *Paying the Hospital in Canada* (New York: Columbia University, Center for the Social Sciences, Nov. 1980), chaps. 6 and 7. Another helpful source is a McKinsey and Company Report, *What Can State and Regional Health Planners Learn from the Canadian Experience in Regulating Hospital Services?* (Washington, D.C.: U.S. Department of Commerce, National Technical Information Service, 1978, HRP-0901082).

18. G. Desrochers, "Le financement des établissements de santé et de services sociaux" *Canadian Public Administration*, 22, 3 (1979), 366–379.

19. W. Glaser, *Paying the Hospital in Canada*, chap. 7, p. 7.

20. S. Lee, "Managing the Health System: Québec Style," *Health Management Forum* (Autumn 1980), 11.

21. For more detail on this method, see J. M. Lance and A. P. Contandriopoulos, "Le regroupement des hôpitaux selon leur production: base d'évaluation de leur Performance," *L'Actualité Economique*, April–June, 1980.

22. W. Glaser, *Paying the Hospital in Canada*, p. 29.

23. McKinsey and Company, *What Can State and Regional Health Planners Learn*, p. 7.

24. W. Glaser, *Paying the Hospital in Canada*.

25. *Cadre de référence pour l'adaptation des ressources aux priorités: plan de développement des ressources en santé* (Québec: Ministère des Affaires Sociales, July 1976).

26. N. Bergeron and A. Couture, *Estimation de l'impact du port obligatoire de la ceinture de sécurité sur les coûts des services de santé au Québec*

(Québec: Ministère des Affaires Sociales, Direction de la Planification des Services de Santé, January 1976).

27. *Guide d'allocation des ressources: services spécialisés et ultra-spécialisés* (Québec: Ministère des Affaires Sociales, August 1978).

28. *L'annuaire du Québec* (Québec: Bureau Statistique du Québec, 1979—1980), chap. 4.

29. For a more detailed discussion of the problems of occupational health in Québec, see *Santé et sécurité au travail: politique Québecoise de la santé et de la sécurité des travailleurs* (Québec: Gouvernement du Québec, Ministère du Développement Social, 1978).

30. *La Presse* (August 4, 1977).

31. Speaking in French, Lévesque said that it was necessary to "*réévaluer en profondeur*" the CLSCs. *La Presse* (October 17, 1978).

32. These data are from "Les CLSCs 5 ans après: pour un bilan." l'information, Anjou, Québec: La Fédération des CLSCs du Québec 1, 4 (1977).

33. Speech before a meeting of the Federation of CLSCs of Québec, October 1977, cited by F. Lesemann, *Du pain et des services: la réforme de la santé et des services sociaux au Québec* (Laval, Québec: Editions Coopératives Albert Saint Martin, 1981), p. 223.

34. Ibid.

35. J. Boutin and J. Bisson, *Les consommateurs et les coûts de la santé au Québec de 1971 à 1975* (Québec: Régie de l'Assurance Maladie, Service de la Recherche et des Statistiques, January 1977).

36. A. Contandriopoulos, "Stimulants économiques et utilisation des services médicaux" *L'Actualité Economique*, April—June, 1980.

37. *Effet des modifications à l'entente sur la dispensation des injections de substance sclérosante* (Québec: Régie d'Assurance Maladie, Service de la Recherche et des Statistiques, August 1976).

38. *Le système des honoraires modulés. rapport du comité sur la rémunération des professionnels de la santé du Québec* (Québec: Ministère des Affaires Sociales, March 1980).

39. Ibid., p. 155. , my translation.

40. *L'annuaire du Québec*, table 28.

41. *Les affaires sociales au Québec* (Québec: Gouvernement du Québec, 1980), p. 119.

42. *Eléments pour une politique de décentralisation administrative*, see n. 16.

43. Ibid.

44. See, e.g., G. Desrochers, "La décentralisation des activités publiques," in C. Tilquin, ed., *Systems Science in Health Care* (Ottawa: Pergamon Press, 1981).

45. M. Renaud, "Québec's New Middle Class." For more recent reflections on this theme, see M. Renaud, "Québec: les aventures d'un Etat narcissique," in J. de Kervasdoué, J. Kimberly, and V. Rodwin, eds., *La*

santé rationnée: la fin d'un mirage (Paris: Economica, 1981).

46. J. Benjamin, *Planification et Politique au Québec* (Montréal: Les Presses de l'Université de Montréal, 1974), p. 114; cited by Renaud, "Québec's New Middle Class."

47. M. Renaud, "Québec's New Middle Class," p. 29.

48. It should be noted that group practice was already growing long before CLSCs were established. It would be misleading to suggest that polyclinics were created only to counterbalance the competition of CLSCs. It seems reasonable, however, to suggest that the growth of CLSCs reinforced the trend toward group practice settings in the delivery of medical care.

49. P. Enterline et al., "The Distribution of Medical Services Before and After 'Free' Medical Care: The Québec Experience," *New England Journal of Medicine* 289 (November 1973), 1174–1178. For a review of Québec's experience with health insurance, see A. McDonald, J. McDonald, and P. Enterline, "Etudes sur l'assurance maladie du Québec," in *Sociologie et Société*, vol. 9. Also see *Responses of Canadian Physicians to the Introduction of Universal Medical Care Insurance: The First Five Years in Québec* (Princeton, N. J.: Mathematica Policy Research, 1980). Available in NCHSR Research Digest Series (Washington, D.C.: DHEW Pub. No. PHS 80-3229). For a recent analysis of the impact of health insurance in Montreal—one that accounts for differential utilization resulting from different health status—see J. Siemiatycki, L. Richardson, and I. Pless, "Equality in Medical Care under National Health Insurance in Montreal," *New England Journal of Medicine* 303 (July 3, 1980), 10–15.

50. L. Bozzini and A. Contandriopoulos, "La pratique médicale au Québec: mythes et réalités," *Sociologie et Société* 9, 1 (April 1977); and J. Brunet, "Priorités dans le domaine de la santé au Québec," speech of the Undersecretary of Social Affairs presented to a Multidisciplinary Conference on Health organized by the journal, *Critère*. (Centre d'Art d'Orford, June 6, 1976).

51. *Le système des honoraires modulés.*

7. HEALTH PLANNING IN A NATIONAL HEALTH SERVICE: ENGLAND

1. DHSS, *The NHS Planning System* (London: Her Majesty's Stationery Office [HMSO], June 1976).

2. B. Abel-Smith, *National Health Service: The First Thirty Years* (London: HMSO, 1978), p. 14.

3. Cited by M. Buxton and R. Klein, "Allocating Health Resources: A Commentary on the Report of the Resource Allocation Working Party," Research Paper No. 3, Royal Commission on the National Health Service (London: HMSO, 1978), p. 1.

4. H. Eckstein, "Planning: A Case Study," *Political Studies* IV (1965), 46–60.

5. G. Maddox, "Muddling Through: Planning for Health Care in England," *Medical Care*, 9, 5 (1971).

6. Abel-Smith, *National Health Service*, pp. 12–13.

7. R. Klein, "The Political Economy of National Health," *The Public Interest* no. 26 (Winter 1972), pp. 112–125.

8. B. Abel-Smith, *National Health Service*, p. 19.

9. H. Eckstein, *The English National Health Service: Its Origins, Structure and Achievement* (Cambridge: Harvard University Press, 1959), p. 236.

10. B. Abel-Smith, *National Health Service*, p. 19.

11. *A Hospital Plan for England and Wales*, Command No. 1604 (London: HMSO, 1962).

12. *The Times*, January 4, 1962; cited by D. Allen, *Hospital Planning: The Development of the 1962 Hospital Plan: A Case Study in Decision Making* (Kent: Pitman Medical Publishing Co., 1979), p. 65.

13. B. Abel-Smith, *National Health Service*, pp. 20, 53.

14. M. Cooper, *Rationing Health Care* (New York: John Wiley & Sons, 1975), p. 61.

15. Ibid., p. 62.

16. B. Abel-Smith, *National Health Service*, p. 25.

17. Ibid.

18. For a thorough analysis of this policy, see J. Butler et al., *Family Doctors and Public Policy* (London: Routledge and Kegan Paul, 1973).

19. D. Macmillan, "The Role of Regional Authorities in Health Planning in Great Britain," in C. Altenstetter, *Changing National-Subnational Relations in Health: Opportunities and Constraints.* (Washington, D.C.: DHEW Pub. No. [NIH] 78–182, 1976), p. 235.

20. M. Cooper, "Health Costs and Expenditures in the United Kingdom," in T. Hu, *International Health Costs and Expenditures* (Washington, D.C.: DHEW Pub. No. [NIH] 76–1067, 1976).

21. M. Buxton and R. Klein, "Allocating Health Resources," p. 2.

22. M. Cooper, *Rationing Health Care*, p. 10.

23. For further details on the Reorganization of 1974, see *Management Arrangements for the Reorganized National Health Service* (London: HMSO, 1972). For further analysis of the reorganization, see R. Brown, *Reorganizing the National Health Service* (Oxford: Blackwell and Robertson, 1979); K. Barnard and K. Lee, eds., *NHS Reorganization: Issues and Prospects* (Leeds: University of Leeds, Nuffield Centre for Health Services Studies, 1974); and R. Levitt, *The Reorganized National Health Service* (London: Croom Helm, 1976).

24. B. Watkins, "Themes in Health Care Planning: A Consideration of the NHS Interim Planning System," University of Manchester: Department of Social Administration, January 1976. Mimeo.

25. R. Brown, *Reorganizing the National Health Service*, p. 36.

26. Cash limits were first officially imposed in 1975 and led to a series of problems. Successive governments failed to build into the limits sufficient funds to cover pay increases and price inflation on the goods purchased by the NHS. As a consequence, health authorities have had to enforce the incomes policy suggested by the government or to proceed with cutbacks in planned improvements. See, e.g., *Report of the TUC Conference to Mark the 30th Anniversary of the Establishment of the NHS* (London: Trade Union Congress, June 29, 1978).

27. See, e.g., DHSS Health Circular (HC) (78)12. It is divided into seven parts. Part I (Taking Stock) examines current planning issues in 1978 and what can be realistically accomplished by the end of the planning period. Part II (Priorities) elaborates issues raised in the Priorities Document of 1976. Part III (Future Developments) projects the state of these issues in the future. Part IV (The National Programme Budget) provides national budgetary figures reflecting the extent to which the priorities will be implemented in the coming year. Part V (Planning Report and Tasks) analyzes a sample of local plans and evaluates them in a national context. Part VI (NHS Manpower Assumptions) calls for an improved information base for each RHA as a prerequisite for future manpower planning. Part VII (NHS Resource Assumptions for Planning Purposes) provides the projected capital and expenditure allocations by RHA.

28. For a full description of joint care planning and financing, see DHSS Health Circulars HC76(18) and HC(77)17 as well as Local Authority Circulars LAC (76)6 and LAC(77)10.

29. T. Booth, *Joint Care Planning: A Case Study of Collaboration Between the Health and Social Services* (Sheffield: University of Sheffield, April 1980), p. 77.

30. C. Graham and M. Fairey, "Health Planning Methods in England," in *Health Planning Methods: Case Studies from the 1978 International Workshop Part II* (Washington, D.C.: DHSS Pub. No. HRP-0250201, pt. 2, 1980).

31. M. Butts, D. Irving, and C. Whitt, *From Principles to Practice: A Commentary on Health Service Planning and Resource Allocation in England from 1970 to 1980* (London: Nuffield Provincial Hospitals Trust [NPHT], 1981), p. 44.

32. W. Glaser, *Paying the Hospital in England* (New York: Columbia University, Center for the Social Sciences, June 1981), p. IV-15.

33. J. Perrin, *Management of Financial Resources in the National Health Service*, Research Paper No. 2, Royal Commission on the National Health Service (London: HMSO, 1978), p. 198.

34. DHSS, *Priorities for Health and Personal Health Services: A Consultative Document* (London: HMSO, 1976).

35. DHSS, *Sharing Resources for Health in England: Report of the Resource Allocation Working Party* (London: HMSO, 1976).

36. *Priorities Document*, p. 1.

37. DHSS, *The Way Forward* (London: HMSO, Sept. 1977), p. 1.

38. P. Fox, "Managing Health Resources, English Style," in G. McLachlan, ed., *By Guess or By What: Information Without Design in the NHS* (Oxford: NPHT, 1978).

39. D. Black, ed., *Inequalities in Health: Report of the Working Group on Inequalities* (London: DHSS, August 1980). This report was written at the initiative of the Labor government when David Ennals was secretary of state for social services. Since it was completed under the Thatcher government, however, it was neither endorsed by the new secretary for social services, Patrick Jenkin, nor published by HMSO. Needless to say, this 417-page, $20 document is very critical of the success of the NHS in promoting equality in health resource provision. In the foreword, Jenkin summarized the report, "It will come as a disappointment to many that over long periods since the inception of the NHS there is generally little sign of health inequalities in Britain diminishing and, in some cases, they may be increasing." This report provides both a thorough review of the literature on inequalities in health and a careful empirical analysis of these inequalities in England as well as in other countries. Another provocative book on this theme, in the English context, is by V. Walters, *Class Inequality and Health Care* (London: Croon Helm, 1980).

40. R. Klein, "Priorities and the Problems of Planning," *British Medical Journal* (October 22, 1977), p. 1097.

41. *Sharing Resources for Health in England*, p. 7.

42. For a thorough analysis of the problems involved in making the concept of equity operational and for an evaluation of the hospital revenue allocation formula in this light, see P. West, "Allocation and Equity in the Public Sector: The Hospital Revenue Allocation Formula," *Applied Economics* 5 (1973), 153–166.

43. M. Buxton and R. Klein, "Distribution of Hospital Provision: Policy Themes and Resource Variations," *British Medical Journal* (February 8, 1975), pp. 345–349.

44. In English parlance, operating expenditures are referred to as revenue.

45. M. Buxton and R. Klein, "Allocating Health Resources." See table 3, p. 26.

46. On this theme, see ibid.

47. A. Barr and R. Logan, "Policy Alternatives for Resource Allocation," *The Lancet* 1 (1977), 994–997.

48. S. Palmer, P. West, and P. Dodd, "Randomness in the RAWP Formula: The Reliability of Mortality Data in the Allocation of National Health Service Revenue," *Journal of Epidemiology and Community Health* 34 (1980), 212–216.

49. M. Buxton and R. Klein, "Allocating Health Resources."

50. S. Senn and H. Shaw, "Resource Allocation: Some Problems in

Applying the National Formula of Area and District Revenue Allocations," *Journal of Epidemiology and Community Health* 32 (1978), 22—27.

51. R. Klein and M. Buxton, "Population Characteristics and the Distribution of General Medical Practitioners," *British Medical Journal* 1 (1979), 463—466.

52. The Working Group on Inequalities in Health under the chairmanship of Sir Douglas Black made a similar point in the following terms: "Where the Working Party (RAWP) have less to say is first in accepting the current distribution of resources as between in-patient and community services, and second in accepting present national rates of utilization of different types of service. What happens is not a good measure of what should happen, however convenient that may be. However, an ideal allocation of resources cannot easily be defined and to us it seems possible only to give some preliminary indications of the steps that can be taken . . . to incorporate shifts between services and changes in the patterns of utilization of services, along with the shifts implied by the RAWP analysis, that may be required. . . . We seek to make two points: first, that policy priorities . . . can be related much more exactly to the needs for health care than has been appreciated; and that only by insisting on such a process of reasoning is it possible to produce, over a period of years, the necessary resources to make a sufficient contribution to the reduction of inequalities in health." (London: DHSS, 1980), p. 248. Also see p. 264.

53. A. Creese et al., "NHS Priorities and RAWP," *British Medical Journal* (November 18, 1978).

54. For further analysis of RAWP principles, see C. Whitt's analysis in M. Butts, D. Irving, and C. Whitt, *From Principles to Practice.*

55. As noted in the RAWP Report, "Resource allocation is concerned with the distribution of financial resources which are used for the provision of real resources. In this sense it is concerned with the means rather than the end. We have not regarded our remit as being concerned with how the resources are deployed. This must be a matter for the administering Authorities and is essentially part of their policy-making, planning and decision-making functions in response to central guidelines on national policies and priorities." p. 8.

56. M. Buxton and R. Klein, "Distribution of Hospital Provisions."

57. This table is based on figures provided by R. Longfield, Finance Division, DHSS, in March 1981.

58. Press Release, DHSS, February 9, 1981.

59. "Third Report from the Social Services Committee," Session 1979—1980, II, 59—60.

60. J. Yudkin, "Changing Patterns of Resource Allocation in a London Teaching District," *British Medical Journal* (October 28, 1978).

61. T. Rathwell, "The Politics of Persuasion" in *The Times Health Supplement* (London: Dec. 12, 1981).

62. C. Davies, "Hospital Centered Health Care: Policies and Politics

in the NHS," in P. Atkinson, et al., eds., *Prospects for the National Health* (London: Croon Helm, 1979).

63. J. Ashford and M. Butts, "Resource Allocation and Planning: The Case for Closer Coordination," in *Resource Allocation and General Policy in the National Health Service* (London: Nuffield Provincial Hospitals Trust, December 1978).

64. *Royal Commission on the National Health Service*, (London: HMSO, 1979), p. 56. The citation is from *Ninth Report from the Expenditure Committee Session 1976/77*, ch. V (London: HMSO, 1977), p. vi.

65. Since this chapter was written, the 1982 administrative reorganization of the NHS eliminated the 90 AHAs leaving day to day management in the hands of 192 district health authorities (DHAs). The purpose of this reform, originally proposed in the consultative document on reorganization, *Patients First* (London: HMSO, 1979), was to reduce administrative costs and increase management responsibilities at the local level. There are likely to be difficult problems, however, under the new arrangements. What will happen, for instance, to the principle of parliamentary responsibility? The NHS remains centrally financed and the secretary of state of the DHSS is still responsible to Parliament for everything that occurs in the NHS. Under the new arrangements, the hospital becomes the cornerstone of a DHA and the FPCs and LAs become administratively more remote. This raises questions as to how strategic health plans to alter resource allocation will be implemented and whether RHAs will distribute finance to DHAs on the basis of local plans or on the basis of central criteria emanating from the DHSS? In short, the problem of linking planning and financing will still need to be addressed.

For a more extensive evaluation of the new administrative arrangements, see *Patients First—Intentions and Consequences: a commentary on the consultative paper on the structure and management of the National Health Service in England and Wales* (Leeds: University of Leeds, Nuffield Centre for Health Services Studies, 1980). For a more general evaluation of health planning in the NHS, which deals with the new administrative arrangements as well as other issues, see K. Barnard, K. Lee, A. Mills, and J. Reynolds, "NHS Planning: An Assessment"—a short paper based on a large study (Leeds: Nuffield Centre).

8. HEALTH PLANNING AMERICAN STYLE

1. S. Axelrod, A. Donabedian, D. Gentry, *Medical Care Chartbook* (Ann Arbor: University of Michigan, 1976); K. Davis, "Equal Treatment and Unequal Benefits: The Medicare Program," *Milbank Memorial Fund Q.* 53 (Fall, 1975), 449–488. Inequities are, of course, not limited to access. They also apply to indicators of outcome. The poor (with family incomes less than $6,000) are sicker than those with family incomes over

$6,000 e.g., with regard to such outcome measures as days of "bed disability" or "restricted activity." Paul Newacheck, Lewis Butler, et al., have found that about 75% of the gap in restricted activity days and bed disability days between the poor and the "nonpoor" is attributable to greater prevalence and severity of activity-limiting chronic conditions most of which are not covered by Medicare and Medicaid. See their "Income and Illness," *Medical Care* 18, 12 (1980), 1165—1176.

2. R. Roemer, C. Kramer, and J. Frink, eds., *Planning Urban Health Services: From Jungle to System* (New York: Springer, 1975).

3. J. Wennberg and A. Gittelsohn, "Small Area Variations in Health Care Delivery," *Science,* 182 (1973). Also see their "Variations in Medical Care Among Small Areas," *Scientific American,* 246 (1982), 120—134.

4. See, e.g., *Priorities for the Use of Resources in Medicine* (Washington, D.C.: Fogarty International Center Proceedings, no. 40, DHEW Publication No. (NIH)77-1288, 1976).

5. The figure for 1965 is from R. Gibson and D. Waldo, "National Health Expenditures, 1980," *Health Care Financing Rev.* (Washington, D.C.: Health Care Financing Administration, September 1981). The figure for 1981 is from D. Waldo, *Health Care Financing Trends* 3, 1 (Washington, D.C.: HCFA, June 1982).

6. R. Gibson and D. Waldo, "National Health Expenditures, 1980," p. 38, table 4.

7. The Hill-Burton Hospital Construction Act was amended in 1949 (P.L. 81-380), 1954 (P.L. 83-483), 1964 (P.L. 88-433), and 1970 (P.L. 91-296). The 1964 amendment added long-term care facilities and expanded the program to include the modernization or replacement of facilities. The 1970 amendment expanded the program to include neighborhood health centers and outpatient facilities in poverty areas and rural communities.

8. Regional Medical Programs were created by Public Law 89-239.

9. P.L. 89-749 (The Comprehensive Health Planning and Public Health Services Amendments).

10. Defining *excess capacity* is a complex and controversial issue. On this topic, see the *National Guidelines for Health Planning* (Washington, D.C.: DHEW publication no. (HRA) 78-643, 1978). Also see R. Berry, Jr., "On Excess Capital Accumulation in the Hospital Industry," Brandeis University Health Policy Consortium, August 1979; W. McClure, *Reducing Excess Capacity* (Excelsior, Minn.: InterStudy, 1976); and Institute of Medicine, *Controlling the Supply of Hospital Beds* (Washington, D.C.: National Academy of Sciences, Oct. 1976).

11. The PSRO Program was enacted as an amendment to the Social Security Act (P.L. 92-603).

12. For a thorough evaluation of the PSRO program, see *Professional Standards Review Organization 1979 Program Evaluation* (Washington, D.C.: U.S. DHSS, Health Care Financing Administration, 1979).

13. Public law 92-603.

14. K. Bauer, "Hospital Rate Setting—This Way to Salvation?" *Milbank Mem. Fund Q.* (Winter 1977).

15. P.L. 93-222.

16. See H. Luft, "How Do Health Maintenance Organizations Achieve Their 'Savings'?" *New England Journal of Medicine* 298 (1978).

17. There are two important qualifications to these points. First, the firm is only required to offer the HMO option if the HMO formally requests it to do so. Second, HMOs are not required to enroll more than 5 percent of their total members during the open enrollment periods.

18. P. L. 93-641, Section 2, January 4, 1975.

19. E. Rubel, "Health Planning and Rate Review," in F. Sattler, ed., *Health Planning and Rate Review: An Integrated Approach to Moderating the Rise in Health Care Costs* (Minneapolis: Interstudy, June 1976).

20. H. J. Sapolsky, "Bottoms Up Is Upside Down," in *Health Planning in the United States: Selected Policy Issues* (Washington, D.C.: National Academy Press, 1981), Vol. II.

21. K. Bauer, *Cost Containment Under P.L. 93-641: Strengthening the Partnership Between Health Planning and Regulation. Final Report* (Cambridge, Mass.: Harvard Center for Community Health and Medical Care, January 1978), p. 29.

22. P.L. 93-641, Section 1526.

23. Social Security Amendments (P.L. 92-603, Section 222); The Health Maintenance Act (P.L. 93-222); Hospital Cost Containment Bill of 1977 (H.R. 6575).

24. For an overall evaluation of the National Health Planning and Resources Development Act, see the studies by the National Institute of Medicine, *Health Planning in the United States: Selected Policy Issues* (Washington, D.C.: National Academy Press, 1981), Vols. I and II; *Health Planning in the United States: Issues in Guideline Development* (Washington, D.C.: National Academy of Sciences, 1980). See also H. Klarman, "Health Planning: Progress, Prospects and Issues," *Milbank Mem. Fund Q.* 56 (1978); and H. Foley, "Health Planning—Demise or Reformation?" *New England Journal of Medicine* 304 (April 16, 1981).

25. T. Marmor and J. Marone, "Representing Consumer Interests: Imbalanced Markets, Health Planning, and the HSAs," in J. McKinlay *Politics and Health Care* (Milbank Reader 6), (Cambridge: MIT Press, 1981).

26. B. Checkaway, "Consumerism in Health Planning Agencies," in *Health Planning in the United States*, Vol. II; B. Vladeck, "Interest-Group Representation and the HSAs: Health Planning and Political Theory," *American Journal of Public Health* 67 (January 1977).

27. L. Butler et al., *Cooperation Between Health Systems Agencies and Professional Standards Review Organizations* (Report to the U.S. DHEW) (San Francisco: Institute for Health Policy Studies, 1976).

28. D. Cohodes, "Interstate Variation in Certificate of Need Programs: A Review and Prospectus," in *Health Planning in the United States*, Vol. II; D. Salkever and T. Bice, "The Impact of Certificate-of-Need Controls on Hospital Investment, *Milbank Memorial Fund Q.* (Spring 1976). Also see Lewin and Associates, *Evaluation of the Efficiency and Effectiveness of the Section 1122 Review Process.* Prepared for the Health Resources Administration, 1975. Distributed by NTIS, U.S. Dept. of Commerce, Washington, D.C.; F. Sloan and B. Steinwald, "Effects of Regulation on Hospital Costs and Use," *Journal of Law and Economics* 81 (1980); K. McCaffree and T. Bice, "The Impact of Capital Expenditure Controls on Health Care Institutions," in D. Hough and G. Misek, eds., *Socioeconomic Issues of Health 1980* (Monroe, Wis.: American Medical Association). A recent article suggests that some of the above studies may be misleading and presents evidence that the growth of hospital costs has been less rapid in those states with rate-setting programs. See B. Biles, C. Schramm, and J. Atkinson "Hospital Cost Inflation under State Rate-Setting Programs," *New England Journal of Medicine* 303 (1980), 664—667.

29. P.L. 96-791. For a good discussion of the possible implications of P.L. 96-791 for HSAs, see D. Helms, "Planning and the Challenge to Promote Competition: How Agencies Can Respond to this New Mandate" (Washington, D.C.: Alpha Center for Health Planning, November 1980); and J. Needleman, "Promoting Competition as a Regulatory Strategy: (Washington, D.C.: Alpha Center for Health Planning, June 1980).

30. Ibid.

31. Report of the House Committee on Interstate and Foreign Commerce on the Health Planning and Resources Development Act of 1979 (H.R. 3917). House Report No. 96-190, Ninety-Sixth Congress, First Session, May 15, 1979, pp. 53—54.

32. The following five bills were introduced following the failure of the Carter administration's 1979 Hospital Cost Containment Act: (1) The National Health Care Reform Act (H.R. 7527); introduced in June 1980 by Congressmen Richard Gephardt and David Stockman; (2) The Health Incentives Reform Act (S. 1485); introduced in July 1979 by Senator David Durenberger; (3) The Health Cost Restraint Act (H.R. 5740); introduced in October 1979 by Congressman Al Ullman; (4) The Comprehensive Health Care Reform Act (S. 1590); introduced in July 1979 by Senator Richard Schweiker; (5) The Consumer Health Expenses Control Act (H.R. 7528); introduced in June 1980 by Congressman James Jones.

33. P. Ellwood, "The Importance of the Market," *J. of Health Policy, Politics and Law* 2 (Winter 1978). P. Ellwood et al., "Competition: Medicine's Creeping Revolution," paper presented at the Sixth Private Sector Conference, March 23, 1981; C. Havighurst, "Role of Competition in Cost Containment," in W. Greenberg, ed., *Competition in the Health Care*

Sector (Germantown, Md.: Aspen Systems Corporation, 1978); C. Havighurst, "Competition in Health Services: Overview, Issues and Answers," *Vanderbilt Law Rev.* 34, 4 (1981); W. McClure, "Broadening the Definition of a Competitive Health Care System" and "Implementing a Competitive System," *Journal of Health Politics, Policy and Law* 3 (1978) and 1 (1982); J. Christianson and W. McClure, "Competition in the Delivery of Medical Care," *New England Journal of Medicine* 301 (October 11, 1979). A. Enthoven, *Health Plan: The Only Practical Solution to the Soaring Cost of Medical Care* (Reading, Mass.: Addison-Wesley Publishing Company, 1980). A revised version of the original Enthoven proposal to Secretary Califano was published in the *New England Journal of Medicine* 298, 12 (1978), under the title "Consumer-Choice Health Plan." Three major journals have recently organized special issues on competition and regulation: *Milbank Memorial Fund Q.* 59, 2 (1981); *Journal of Health Politics, Policy and Law* 7, 1 (1981); *Vanderbilt Law Review* 34, 4 (1981).

34. A. Enthoven, *Health Plan*.

35. L. Butler et al., *Medical Life on the Western Frontier: The Competitive Impact of Prepaid Medical Care Plans in California.* Berkeley: Institute of Governmental Studies. Also, see H. Luft, "On the Potential Failure of Good Ideas: An Interview with the Originator of Murphy's Law," *Journal of Health Politics, Policy and Law* 17, 1 (Spring, 1982), 45—53.

36. A. Enthoven, "The Competition Strategy: Status and Prospects," *New England Journal of Medicine* 304 (January 8, 1981), 111.

37. A. Enthoven, *Health Plan*, p. 96.

38. S. Altman and S. Weiner, "Regulation as a Second Best," in W. Greenberg, ed., *Competition in the Health Care Sector*, p. 351.

39. S. Schroeder and J. Showstack, "Financial Incentives to Perform Medical Procedures and Laboratory Tests: Illustrative Models of Office Practice," *Medical Care* 16 (April 1978) 289—298; M. Blumberg, "Rational Provider Prices: An Incentive for Improved Health Delivery," in C. Chacko, ed., *Health Handbook—1978* (Amsterdam: North Holland Publishing Company, 1978).

40. Cited in "Impact," DHEW Region VIII Health Planning Newsletter, PACT Health Planning Center, Denver, Col., vol. 2, no. 10, 1978.

41. P. Ruderman, "The Political Economy of Fee-Setting and the Future of Fee-for-Service," in R. Fraser, ed., *Health Economics Symposium: Proceedings of the First Canadian Conference, September 4—6, 1974* (Kingstone, Canada: Industrial Relations Center, Queens University, 1976).

42. D. Altman, *Connections Between Hospital Rate Setting and Planning in Maryland and Rhode Island* (Harvard Center for Community Health and Medical Care, June 1976).

43. H. Cohen, "Experience of A State Cost Control Commission," in M. Zubkoff, I. Raskin, and R. Hanft, eds., *Hospital Cost Containment:*

Selected Notes for Future Policy (New York: Prodist, 1978).

44. M. Sweetland, D. Altman, and W. Motter, *Institutional Responses to Evolving Health Planning and Regulatory Programs: Case Studies From Two New England States* (Harvard Center for Community Health and Medical Care, January 1978); R. Evans, *Linkages Between Planning, Regulation and Rate Setting in New Jersey: The Case of a Perinatal Care Center Designation* (Harvard Center for Community Health and Medical Care (January 1978); and J. Brown, *Facility Expansion and Facility Closure: Two Case Studies in Health Planning and Regulation from Rochester, New York* (Harvard University Center for Community Health and Medical Care, January 1978).

45. J. Iglehart, "New Jersey's Experiment with DRG-Based Hospital Reimbursement," *New England Journal of Medicine* (December 23, 1982). Also, see the four-volume evaluation published by the Health Research and Educational Trust (Rocky Hill, N.J., 08553).

46. N. Hollander, "Linking Health Planning and Reimbursement: Blue Cross Organization Experiences," paper delivered at the Annual Meeting of the American Public Health Association, Washington, D.C.: October 31, 1977.

47. H. Blum, *Expanding Health Care Horizons: From a General Systems Concept of Health to a National Health Policy* (Oakland, Calif.: Third Party Associates, 1976). See chapter written with J. Showstack.

48. This is one of the main points in a critique of A. Enthoven's proposal by E. Ginsberg, "The Competitive Solution: Two Views," *New England Journal of Medicine* (November 6, 1980).

49. For a comprehensive review of the impact of these policy shifts, see P. Lee, C. Estes, L. Leroy, and R. Newcomber, "Health Policy and the Aged," *Annual Review of Gerontology and Geriatrics* 3 (1982).

50. These issues are discussed in more detail in J. de Kervasdoué, J. Kimberly, and V. Rodwin, eds., *The End of An Illusion: The Future of Health Policy in Western Industrialized Nations* (Berkeley, Los Angeles, London: University of California Press, 1984).

9. COMPARISONS AND INTERPRETATIONS

1. The CNPF would like to make people "responsible for their own health." Personal interview with M. Vandermelen, representative of the *Confédération Nationale du Patronat Français* (CNPF) on the Board of Directors of the National Health Insurance Fund (CNAMTS).

2. *Gouvernement du Québec, Santé et Sécurité au Travail,* 1978; and DHSS, *Priorities for Health and Personal Health Services: A Consultative Document.* (London: Her Majesty's Stationary Office, 1976).

3. A. Wildavsky, "Can Health Be Planned?" Michael Davis lecture,

Center for Health Administration, Graduate School of Business, University of Chicago, 1976.

4. J. de Kervasdoué, "Les politiques de santé sont-elles adaptées à la pratique médicale?" *Sociologie du Travail* 3 (1979).

5. A. Wildavsky, "Doing Better and Feeling Worse: The Political Pathology of Health Policy," *Daedalus* (Winter 1977), pp. 122–123.

6. M. Webber and H. Rittel, "Dilemmas in a General Theory of Planning," *Policy Sciences* 4 (1973), 155–169.

7. Ibid.

8. A. Wildavsky, "Can Health Be Planned?" p. 7.

9. J. de Kervasdoué, "Les politiques de santé," p. 254.

10. R. Alford, *Health Care Politics* (Chicago: University of Chicago Press, 1975), p. xiv.

11. Classic examples of this approach may be found in R. Dahl, *Who Governs?* and N. Polsby, *Community Power and Political Theory* (New Haven: Yale University Press, 1961 and 1963). Also see A. Wildavsky, *The Politics of the Budgetary Process*, 2d ed. (Boston: Little, Brown and Co., 1974).

12. R. Klein and C. Davies, "Britain: Possible Futures for the NHS," in J. de Kervasdoué, J. Kimberly, and V. Rodwin, *The End of An Illusion: The Future of Health Policy in Western Industrialized Nations* (Berkeley, Los Angeles, London: University of California Press, 1984). For further elaboration on the notion of "corporate stalemate," see R. Klein, "The Corporate State, the Health Service and the Professions," *N.U.Q.* (Spring 1977). For a more general interpretation of the "new corporatism," see H. Wilensky, *The "New Corporatism," Centralization, and the Welfare State* (Beverly Hills: Sage Publications, 1976).

13. T. Lowi, "American Business, Public Policy, Case Studies, and Political Theory," *World Politics: A Quarterly Journal of International Relations* 16, 4 (1964), 681.

14. R. Friedland, "Introduction" to Special Issue on "State Intervention and the Social Wage: The Politics of Social Services Expansion," *International Journal of Health Services* 9, 2 (1979), 196.

15. T. Marmor, D. Wittman, and T. Heagy, "The Politics of Medical Inflation," *Journal of Health Politics, Policy and Law* 1 (1975), 73.

16. R. Alford, *Health Care Politics*, p. 251.

17. Ibid.

18. Ibid.

19. Ibid.

20. Ibid.

21. M. Renaud, "On the Structural Constraints to State Intervention in Health," *Int. J. of Health Services* 5, 4 (1975), 559–571.

22. Ibid., p. 559.

23. Ibid., p. 565.

24. J. O'Connor, *The Fiscal Crisis of the State* (New York: St. Martin's Press, 1973), p. 6.

25. C. Offe, "Structural Problems of the Capitalist State," in K. von Beyme, ed., *German Political Studies* (London: Russell Sage, 1974), p. 247.

26. M. Renaud, "Réforme ou illusion: une analyse des interventions de l'Etat Québecois dans le domaine de la santé," *Sociologie et Sociétés* 9, 1 (1977), 127–152.

27. M. Renaud, "Structural Constraints," p. 568.

28. Ibid.

29. Ibid.

30. Ibid., p. 564.

31. Ibid. p. 564. It is difficult to evaluate on a theoretical level the relationship between the capitalist mode of economic growth and the diseases of civilization because there are so many theories of socialism, none of which explicitly discusses this issue, so far as I know. If Renaud's position is to be evaluated based on the experience of self-proclaimed "socialist" nations, it would not stand up. In this regard, he wisely refrains from citing any evidence based on the Soviet experience. His citations on China are inappropriate because they do not address the relationship between socialism and diseases of civilization.

32. C. Offe, "The Theory of the Capitalist State and the Problem of Policy Formation," in L. Lindberg et al., *Stress and Contradiction*, 125–144. Also see V. Navarro's development of these ideas in *Medicine Under Capitalism* (New York: Prodist, 1976), part IV.

33. On the theme of citizen participation in health planning, see B. Checkoway, ed., *Citizens and Health Care: Participation and Planning for Social Change* (New York: Pergamon Press, 1981).

34. V. Navarro, "Redefining the Health Problem and Implications for Planning Personal Health Services," *HSMHA Health Reports* 86, 8 (1971), pp. 711–724. For a succinct statement on the broadening goals of health planning, also see P. Lee, "The Frontiers of Health Planning," *American Journal of Health Planning* 1, 2 (1976), 1–6.

35. E. Lévy et al., *Economie du système de santé* (Paris: Dunod, 1975); S. Wolfe et al., "The Work of a Group of Doctors in Saskatchewan," *Milbank Mem. Fund Q* 46, 103 (1968); J. Last, "The Iceberg—Completing the Clinical Picture in General Practice," *The Lancet* 7297, 28 (1963); I. Bogatyrev, *Morbidity of Urban Populations and Standards of Therapeutic and Prophylactic Care* (New York: American Public Health Association, 1974).

36. L. Hirshhorn, "Toward a Political Economy of the Service Society," 1974, and "The Social Crisis, Part II: Social Services in the Transition to Post-Industrial Society," 1975. Working papers no. 229 and 252, Institute of Urban and Regional Development, University of California, Berkeley. See sections on health.

37. See, e.g., DHSS, *Prevention is Everybody's Business* (London: Her Majesty's Stationary Office, 1976).

38. G. B. Shaw, *Doctor's Dilemma* (London: Constable, 1930), Preface.

39. The literature on regionalization is vast. For some recent con-

tributions, see C. Altenstetter, ed., *Changing National-Subnational Relations in Health: Opportunities and Constraints* (Washington D. C.: DHEW Publication no. [NIH] 76-1067, 1976).

40. For recent evidence on the effect of regionalization on the quality of surgery, see H. Luft, J. Bunker, and A. Enthoven, "Should Operations Be Regionalized? The Empirical Relation between Surgical Volume and Mortality," *New England Journal of Medicine*, 301 (1979), 1364—1369.

41. Regional disparities in the distribution of Soviet health resources have been documented in some detail: V. Rodwin, "Equal Access and the Distribution of Health Resources: A Study of the Soviet Health Service, A Centrally Planned Regional Health System," Senior thesis (Madison: University of Wisconsin, 1973). For two different perspectives on the Soviet health system, see M. Field, *Soviet Socialized Medicine* (New York: Free Press, 1967); and V. Navarro, *Social Security and Medicine in the USSR* (Lexington, Mass.: D. C. Health, 1977).

42. This point has been made in the case of England by M. Buxton and R. Klein, *Allocating Health Resources: A Commentary on the Report of the Resource Allocation Working Party*, The Royal Commission on the National Health Service (London: HMSO, 1978), p. 4.

43. J. Bradshaw, "A Taxonomy of Social Need," in G. McLachlan, ed., *Problems and Progress in Medical Care* (London: Oxford University Press, 1972).

44. This point is elaborated in H. Blum, *Planning for Health*, 2d ed. (New York: Human Sciences Press, 1981), chap. 4.

45. For further elaboration on the concept of health care rationing, see M. Cooper, *Rationing Health Care* (Toronto: Halstead Press, 1975). H. Luft, "Health Maintenance Organizations and the Rationing of Medical Care," *Milbank Memorial Fund Q.* 60, 2 (1982); and D. Mechanic, "Theories of Rationing," chap. 5 of his *Future Issues in Health Care: Social Policy and the Rationing of Medical Services* (New York: Free Press, 1979); and A. Culyer, "Rationing Health Care Resources: The Second Step in Need Evaluation," chap. 8 in his *Need and the National Health Service* (Oxford: Martin Robertson, 1979).

46. M. Cooper, *Rationing Health Care*.

APPENDIX 1. COMPARATIVE HEALTH SYSTEMS: NOTES ON THE LITERATURE

1. For a thorough introduction to the comparative study of health systems, see R. Elling, *Cross-National Study of Health Systems* (New Brunswick, N. J.: Transaction Books, 1980). For a comprehensive annotated bibliography on this topic, see R. Elling, *Cross-National Study of Health Systems: Concepts, Methods and Data Sources* and *Cross-National Study of Health Systems: Countries, World Regions, and Special Problems* (Detroit: Gale

Research Company, 1980). Also, see the *International Journal of Health Services*; and the Comparative Health Systems Newsletter, Department of Community Medicine, University of Connecticut Health Center, Farmington, CT 06032.

2. For a good example of how anthropologists approach the comparative study of health systems, see C. Leslie, ed., *Theoretical Foundation for the Comparative Study of Medical Systems*, vol. 12 of *Social Science and Medicine* (1978). For a sociological perspective, see R. Elling, *Comparative Health Systems*, supplement to Volume XII, no. 2 of *Inquiry*, 1975. For a political science approach, see C. Altenstetter, ed., *Changing National-Subnational Relations in Health: Opportunities and Constraints* (Washington, D.C.: U.S. DHEW Publication no. (NIH)78-182, 1978). For an economic approach, see T. Hu, ed., *International Health Costs and Expenditures* (Washington, D.C.: U.S. DHEW Publication no. (NIH)76-1067, 1976); and S. Schweitzer, ed., *Policies for the Containment of Health Care Costs and Expenditures* (Washington, D.C.: U.S. DHEW Publication no. (NIH)78-184, 1978).

3. This point has been made by K. Dumbaugh and D. Neuhauser, "International Comparisons of Health Services: Where Are We?" *Social Science and Medicine* 13B (1979), 221–223.

4. See, e.g., J. Corson, *Loiterings in Europe* (New York: Harper, 1848); A. Muhry, *Observations on the Comparative State of Medicine in France, England and Germany* (Philadelphia: A. Waldie, 1838).

5. See, e.g., the *Medical Tribune* (New York: Medical Tribune, Inc.); *Journal Médical des Voyages* (Paris).

6. M. Roemer, *Health Care Systems in World Perspective* (Ann Arbor: Health Administration Press, 1976); J. Fry, *Medicine in Three Societies—Comparison of Medical Care in the USSR, USA and UK* (New York: Elsevier, 1970); I. Douglas-Wilson and G. McLachlan, eds., *Health Service Prospects: An International Survey* (London: Nuffield Provincial Hospitals Trust, 1974); J. Fry and W. Farndale, *International Medical Care: A Comparison and Evaluation of Medical Care Throughout the World* (Wallingord, Pa: Washington Square East, 1972); and V. and R. Sidel, *A Healthy State: An International Perspective on the Crisis in United States Medical Care* (New York: Pantheon, 1977).

7. G. Forsyth, *Doctors and State Medicine: A Study of the British Health Service* (London: Pitman Medical, 1966); A. Lindsey, *Socialized Medicine in England and Wales* (Chapel Hill: University of North Carolina Press, 1962); V. and R. Sidel, *Serve the People: Observations on Medicine in the People's Republic of China* (New York: Josiah Macy, 1973); G. Hyde, *The Soviet Health Service: A Historical and Comparative Study* (London: Lawrence and Wilshardt, 1974); H. Sigerist, *Medicine and Health in the Soviet Union* (New York: Citadel Press, 1947); and R. and J. Weinerman, *Social Medicine in Eastern Europe: Organization of Health Services and the Education of Medical Personnel in Czechoslovakia, Hungary, and Poland* (Cambridge: Harvard University Press, 1969).

8. R. Kohn and K. White, eds., *Health Care: An International Study* (London: Oxford University Press, 1976). Also, see R. Bridgman, *Hospital Utilization: An International Study* (Oxford: Oxford University Press, 1979). R. Maxwell, *Health and Wealth* (Lexington: D. C. Heath, 1981).

9. H. Eckstein, *The English National Health Services: Its Origins, Structure and Achievements* (Cambridge: Harvard University Press, 1959); D. Gill, *The British National Health Service: A Sociologist's Perspective* (Washington, D.C.: DHHS, NIH Publication no. 80-2054, July, 1980); V. Navarro, *Class Struggle, the State and Medicine* (New York: Prodist, 1978); C. Altenstetter, *Health Policy-Making and Administration in Western Germany and the United States* (Beverly Hills: Sage Publications, 1974); D. Stone, *The Limits of Professional Power: National Health Care in the Federal Republic of Germany* (Chicago: University of Chicago Press, 1980); M. Field, *Soviet Socialized Medicine* (New York: Free Press, 1967); V. Navarro, *Social Security and Medicine in the USSR* (Lexington, Mass: D. C. Heath, 1977).

10. R. Elling and H. Kerr, "Selection of Contrasting National Health Systems for In-Depth Study," *Inquiry*, Supplement to vol. 12, 2 (June 1975), 25–40.

11. See H. Teune, "The Logic of Comparative Policy Analysis," and T. Marmor, A. Bridges, and W. Hoffman, "Comparative Politics and Health Policies: Notes on Benefits, Costs, Limits," both in D. Ashford, ed., *Comparing Public Policies* (Beverly Hills: Sage Publications, 1978).

12. See, e.g., T. Litman and L. Robins, "Comparative Analysis of Health Care Systems," *Social Science and Medicine* 5 (1971), 573–581; D. Stone, "Drawing Lessons from Comparative Health Research," in R. Straetz, M. Liberman, and A. Sardell, eds., *Critical Issues in Health Policy* (Lexington: D. C. Heath, 1981); K. White, "International Comparisons of Health Service Systems," *Milbank Memorial Fund Q.* 46 (1968), Part 2, 117–125.

13. O. Anderson, *Health Care: Can There Be Equity? The United States, Sweden, and England* (New York: John Wiley & Sons, 1972).

14. R. Weinerman, "Research on Comparative Health Systems," *Medical Care* 10:3 (1971).

15. O. Anderson, *Health Care: Can There be Equity?* p. 21.

16. M. Field, "The Concept of 'Health System' at the Macrosociological Level," *Social Science and Medicine* 7 (1973), 763.

17. J. De Miguel, "A Framework for the Study of National Health Systems," *Inquiry*, Supplement to vol. 12, 2 (June 1975), 10–24.

18. D. Mechanic, *The Growth of Bureaucratic Medicine* (New York: John Wiley & Sons, 1976), p. 43.

19. M. Field, *Comparative Health Systems: Differentiation and Convergence, Final Report* (Washington, D.C.: National Center for Health Services Research, Grant #HS-00272, 1978). Also see his, "The Health System and the Polity: A Contemporary American Dialectic," *Social Science and Medicine*, 14A (1980), 397–413.

20. M. Field, *Comparative Health Systems*, p. 98.

21. M. Roemer, *Comparative National Policies on Health Care* (New York: Marcel Dekker, 1977); M. and R. Roemer, *Health Care Systems and Comparative Manpower Policies* (New York: Marcel Dekker, 1981); and T. Marmor, A. Bridges, and W. Hoffman, "Comparative Politics and Health Policies."

22. V. Sidel, "International Comparisons of Health Services: How? Who? Why?" in R. Straetz, M. Liberman, and A. Sardell, *Critical Issues in Health Policy*.

23. D. Falcone, "Comparing Comparative Perspectives," *Journal of Health Politics, Policy and Law* 3:1 (1978), 124 – 127.

24. H. D. Banta and K. B. Kemp, eds., *The Management of Health Care Technology in Nine Countries* (New York: Springer Publishing Company, 1982).

25. J. de Kervasdoué, J. Kimberly, and V. Rodwin, eds., *The End of an Illusion; The Future of Health Policy in Western Industrialized Nations* (Berkeley and Los Angeles, London: University of California Press, 1984).

26. G. McLachlan and A. Maynard, *The Public/Private Mix for Health: The Relevance and Effects of Change* (London: Nuffield Provincial Hospitals Trust, 1982).

27. W. Glaser, *Social Settings and Medical Organization: A Cross-National Study of the Hospital* (New York: Atherton Press, 1970).

28. W. Glaser, *Paying the Doctor, Systems of Remuneration and Their Effects* (Baltimore: Johns Hopkins Press, 1970).

29. W. Glaser, *Health Insurance Bargaining: Foreign Lessons for Americans* (New York: Gardner Press, 1978).

30. B. Abel-Smith, *Value for Money in Health Services* (London: Heinemann, 1976); J. Babson, *Health Care Delivery Systems: A Multinational Survey* (London: Pitman Medical, 1972).

31. J. Blanpain, L. Delesie, and H. Nys, *National Health Insurance and Health Resources: The European Experience* (Cambridge: Harvard University Press, 1978).

32. A Blomqvist, *The Health Care Business: International Evidence on Private versus Public Health Care Systems* (Vancouver: The Fraser Institute, 1979).

33. J. Van Langendonck, *Prelude to Harmony on a Community Theme: Health Care Insurance Policies in the Six and Britain* (London: Oxford University Press, 1975).

34. R. Maxwell, *Health Care, The Growing Dilemma: Needs Versus Resources in Western Europe, the U.S. and the U.S.S.R.* (New York: McKinsey and Co., 1974).

35. M. Roemer, *Comparative National Policies on Health Care*; O. Anderson, *Health Care: Can There Be Equity?*; and H. Leichter, *A Comparative Approach to Policy Analysis: Health Care Policy in Four Nations* (Cambridge:

Cambridge University Press, 1979).

36. O. Anderson, "Styles of Planning Health Services: The United States, Sweden, and England," *International Journal of Health Services* I (May 1971); H. Blum, "Does Health Planning Work Anywhere, and If So, Why?" *American Journal of Health Planning* 3, 3 (1978), 34–47; R. Elling, "Health Planning in International Perspective," *Medical Care* 9, 3 (1971); H. Hilleboe, A. Barkuus, and W. Thomas, *Approaches to National Health Planning* (Geneva: WHO, Public Health Papers, No. 46, 1972); and T. Marmor and A. Bridges, "American Planning Concerns and the Lessons of Comparative Experience," *Journal of Health Politics, Policy and Law* 5 (1980).

The international conferences were organized by the U.S. DHEW, the Pan American Health Organization (PAHO), and the World Health Organization (WHO). They have resulted in three publications: H. Blum (rapporteur) *Health Planning: An International View*. Report of an International Workshop, May 31–June 4, 1977, Copenhagen, Denmark (Washington, D.C.: U.S. DHEW, HRA, Bureau of Health Planning, 1977). H. Blum (rapporteur), *Health Planning Methods: An International Perspective* (Washington, D.C.: U.S. DHEW Publication No. HRP-0250101, 1979); and *Health Planning Methods: Case Studies from the 1978 International Workshop. Part I and Part II* (Washington, D.C.: U.S. DHEW Publications No. HRP-0250201 and No. HRP-0250301, 1980).

ACKNOWLEDGMENTS

This book could not have been written without the benefit of extensive conversations with planners, civil servants, doctors, and scholars in France, Québec, England, and the United States. Many of these people have taken the time to react to portions of this manuscript; some have become colleagues and friends.

In France, I am grateful to Dominique Coudreau, Béatrice d'Intignano, Dominique Jolly, Jean de Kervasdoué, Emile Lévy, Gabriel Pallez, Simone Sandier, Jean-Marc Simon, and Jean-Claude Stephan, for their generous assistance. In addition, I owe thanks to Jean-Marc Alby, Pierre Bonamour, the late Robert Bridgman, Marc Douriez, Francis Fagnani, Jacques Hossard, Jean-François Lacronique, Michèlle Liess, Bernard Pissaro, Gérard de Pouvourville, Christian Ramphft, and the late Georges Rösch.

In Québec, I am grateful to Marc Renaud for helping me at every stage of work on the case study and reading numerous drafts. I also owe thanks to Pierre Bergeron, Gilbert Blain, Luciano Bozzini, Jacques Brunet, François Canonne, André-Pierre Contandriopoulos, Gilles DesRochers, Georges Desrosiers, Paul Lamarche, Denis Lazure, Sidney Lee, and Michel Peltier.

In England, I am grateful to Rudolf Klein, Gordon McLachlan, and Tom Rathwell for reading drafts, arranging interviews, and bringing critical documents to my attention. I also owe thanks to Brian Abel-Smith, Keith Barnard, Michael Butts, Celia Davies, Derek Gill, Cliff Graham, Dick Longfield, Mike Lillywhite, Alan Maynard, and Gregory

Parston. Professor Klein as well as the editor of this series, Professor Charles Leslie, read the entire manuscript and made helpful comments throughout.

My colleagues at the Institute for Health Policy Studies, University of California, San Francisco, Ted Benjamin, Sydney Halpern, Susan Maerki, Jon Showstack, and Joan Trauner made helpful improvements in reviewing the chapter on the United States. The same applies for Doctors Henrik Blum and Philip R. Lee. My friends, Richard Bateson, Guilhem Fabre, John Forester, Erland Marcer and particularly Simon Neustein, as well as Marc Rodwin, read or at least discussed with me, drafts of the manuscript and never refrained from pointing out deficiencies, and recommending changes.

Portions of this manuscript were submitted as a doctoral dissertation in the Department of City and Regional Planning, University of California, Berkeley. I am grateful to Professors Henrik Blum and Harold Wilensky for helping immensely during this stage of the project and subsequently, as well. I also appreciate the help of Professors Stephen Cohen, Jack Dyckman, Donald Foley, Richard Meier, and Melvin Webber.

There is one person to whom I am especially indebted— Doctor Philip R. Lee, my mentor since the first day of this project. His vision, enthusiasm, and unflinching support as well as his substantive contributions and painstaking reviews of numerous drafts entitle him to share in whatever praise this book might inspire.

Needless to say, I alone am responsible for possible errors of fact and interpretation.

In the course of this research, I have received financial support from the National Institute of Mental Health, the Institute of International Studies, University of California, Berkeley, and the Council for European Studies. I have also benefited from important institutional support. In France I was based at the Centre de Recherche en Gestion, Ecole Polytechnique, and at the Assistance Publique. At the University of California, Berkeley, I was based at the Institute of

Urban and Regional Development. In 1981, I was a post-doctoral fellow at the Alcohol Research Group (ARG) in Berkeley. I am grateful to Robin Room, Ron Roizen, Larry Wallack, Fried Wittman and other members of ARG for providing a most congenial working environment. In 1982, I was a postdoctoral fellow in the Medical Anthropology Program, the Aging Health Policy Center, and the Institute for Health Policy Studies (IHPS) at the University of California, San Francisco. I am much obliged to Professors Margaret Clark, Carroll Estes, and Philip R. Lee for making these arrangements possible. I also owe thanks to grant funds from the Pew Memorial Trust for health policy research.

Finally, I wish to thank Lynne Stiles for drawing the figures and Paula Brubaker, Eunice Chee, Les Gates, and Cathy Kulka of IHPS for first rate secretarial support.

INDEX

Designer: UC Press Staff
Compositor: Trend Western
Printer: Braun-Brumfield, Inc.
Binder: Braun-Brumfield, Inc.
Text: 11 pt Baskerville
Display: Baskerville/Optima